Rad Tech's Guide to
CT: Imaging Procedures, Patient Care, and Safety

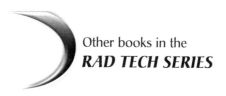

Other books in the
RAD TECH SERIES

Rad Tech's Guide to
CT: Imaging Procedures, Patient Care, and Safety

Deborah Lynn Durham, MA, RT(R), (MR), (CT)
Chairman of CT/MRI Curricula
Forsyth Technical Community College
Advance, North Carolina

Series Editor
Euclid Seeram, RTR, BSc, MSc, FCAMRT
Medical Imaging Advanced Studies
British Columbia Institute of Technology
Burnaby, British Columbia, Canada

b
**Blackwell
Science**

©2002 by Blackwell Science, Inc.

EDITORIAL OFFICES:
Commerce Place, 350 Main Street, Malden, Massachusetts 02148, USA
Osney Mead, Oxford OX2 0EL, England
25 John Street, London WC1N 2BS, England
23 Ainslie Place, Edinburgh EH3 6AJ, Scotland
54 University Street, Carlton, Victoria 3053, Australia

OTHER EDITORIAL OFFICES:
Blackwell Wissenschafts-Verlag GmbH, Kurfürstendamm 57, 10707 Berlin, Germany
Blackwell Science KK, MG Kodenmacho Building, 7-10 Kodenmacho Nihombashi,
   Chuo-ku, Tokyo 104, Japan
Iowa State University Press, A Blackwell Science Company, 2121 S. State Avenue,
   Ames, Iowa 50014-8300, USA

DISTRIBUTORS:
The Americas
   Blackwell Publishing
   c/o AIDC
   P.O. Box 20
   50 Winter Sport Lane
   Williston, VT 05495-0020
   (Telephone orders: 800-216-2522;
      fax orders: 802-864-7626)
Australia
   Blackwell Science Pty, Ltd.
   54 University Street
   Carlton, Victoria 3053
   (Telephone orders: 03-9347-0300;
      fax orders: 03-9349-3016)

Outside The Americas and Australia
   Blackwell Science, Ltd.
   c/o Marston Book Services, Ltd.
   P.O. Box 269
   Abingdon
   Oxon OX14 4YN
   England
   (Telephone orders: 44-01235-465500;
      fax orders: 44-01235-465555)

Acquisitions: Beverly Copland
Development: Julia Casson
Production: GraphCom Corporation
Manufacturing: Lisa Flanagan
Marketing Manager: Toni Fournier
Cover and interior design: Dana Peick, GraphCom Corporation
Typesetting: GraphCom Corporation
Printed and bound by Western Press

Printed in the United States of America
01 02 03 04 5 4 3 2 1

Library of Congress Cataloging-in-Publication Data

Durham, Deborah L.
      Rad tech's guide to CT : imaging procedures, patient care, and safety / by
Deborah Lynn Durham.
      p. ; cm.
      ISBN 0-632-04491-8
      1. Tomography. I. Title: Guide to CT. II. Title.
[DNLM: 1. Tomography, X-Ray Computed—methods—Handbooks. 2. Tomography,
X-Ray Computed—methods—Outlines. 3. Technology, Radiologic—methods—
Handbooks. 4. Technology, Radiologic—methods—Outlines. WN 39 D961r2001]
RC78.7.T6 D8675 2001
616.07'57—dc21

                                                            2001025054

To Jack, my one and only,
and to my two "furry" best friends, Jordie and Chloe

TABLE OF CONTENTS

SERIES EDITOR'S FOREWORD

Blackwell Science's Rad Tech Series in radiologic technology is intended to provide a clear and comprehensive coverage of a wide range of topics and prepare students to write their entry-to-practice registration examination. Additionally, this series can be used by working technologists to review essential and practical concepts and principles and to use them as tools to enhance their daily skills during the examination of patients in the radiology department.

The Rad Tech Series features short books covering the fundamental core curriculum topics for radiologic technologists at both the diploma and the specialty levels, as well as act as knowledge sources for continuing education as defined by the American Registry for Radiologic Technologists (ARRT).

This entry-to-practice series includes books on radiologic physics, equipment operation, patient care, radiographic technique, radiologic procedures, radiation protection, image production and evaluation, and quality control. This specialty series features books on computed tomography (CT)—physics and instrumentation, patient care and safety, and imaging procedures; mammography; and quality management in imaging sciences.

In *Rad Tech's Guide to CT: Imaging Procedures, Patient Care, and Safety*, Deborah Durham, a renowned educator in CT and MRI and department chair of CT and MRI Curricula at Forsyth Technical Community College in North Carolina, presents a clear and concise coverage of patient care and safety issues in CT, as well as CT imaging procedures. Topics include patient care and safety, imaging procedures that describe CT of the head and brain, neck, spine, chest, musculoskeletal system, abdomen, and pelvis.

Debbie Durham has done an excellent job in explaining significant concepts that are mandatory for the successful performance of quality CT in clinical practice. Students, technologists, and educators alike will find this book a worthwhile addition to their libraries.

Enjoy the pages that follow; remember, your patients will benefit from your wisdom.

Euclid Seeram, RTR, BSc, MSc, FCAMRT
Series Editor
British Columbia, Canada

PREFACE

Rad Tech's Guide to CT: Imaging Procedures, Patient Care, and Safety is intended to be a simple and concise guide for CT imaging to enhance the technologist's efficiency and effectiveness in producing a high-quality CT examination. It also is designed to help students prepare for the ARRT CT advanced examination.

The content of two sections of the ARRT CT examination is divided appropriately into chapters. An introduction is provided that outlines the topics for each chapter. Each chapter is then subdivided into specific headings, again based on the examination specifications. Tables are used to make information easy to comprehend and locate, especially topics such as drugs and outcomes, contrast administration, and injection rates. Paragraphs are short and concise for easy reading.

The first chapter discusses patient care and safety. It is written in paragraph style with tables and information presented in a bulleted format. This chapter coincides with the first section of the ARRT specifications; consequently, it is a fairly lengthy chapter.

The second chapter examines the focus of the questions asked about the types of studies in the imaging procedures' section of the ARRT examination. Definitions of terms are provided in paragraph style with the use of tables. The definitions of specific terms are discussed before the different body parts are studied and reviewed. These terms are presented in relation to protocols and anatomy.

Chapters 3 though 9 discuss the seven types of studies performed on specific anatomic parts. These studies are divided into head, neck, chest, abdomen, pelvis, and musculoskeletal system. Each chapter begins with an introduction and table that describe a routine protocol for the type of study. A protocol is a set of parameters used for a specific examination: the technique parameters, how images are reconstructed, and the use of contrast. Protocols used for more specific anatomy in each of the regions are presented. Strategic anatomy is described with tips on localization on CT axial images. Common pathologic conditions in the region, usually diagnosed with CT, are defined.

Rad Tech's Guide to CT: Imaging Procedures, Patient Care, and Safety is constructed as an "easy to find facts" study guide for the ARRT advanced CT examination. It can be used by CT technologists as a study guide for the examination, the passing of which is required for technologists to continue practicing CT technology in all health care facilities. Insurance companies and the public are demanding quality health care in all settings—hospitals, outpatient facilities, or physician offices. *Rad Tech's Guide to CT: Imaging Procedures, Patient Care, and Safety* will serve as a means to acquire quality CT technologists producing quality examinations. It will also serve as a clinical reference guide to enhance the skills of the CT registered technologists, ensuring good quality care.

Rad Tech's Guide to CT: Imaging Procedures, Patient Care, and Safety also serves CT students in their clinical and classroom studies. Laboratory values, drug use, protocol selection, and contrast information will be at their fingertips at all times because of its size, which will also be true for the practicing CT technologist who has already taken the examination but may have difficulty remembering the details and values not used on a daily basis.

Rad Tech's Guide to CT: Imaging Procedures, Patient Care, and Safety will also benefit the radiography student. The ARRT radiography examination has its own set of specifications for testing. Included on this particular examination are questions about CT. The radiography student must also complete a rotation through a CT clinical facility. This reference guide will be an asset in the CT clinical area and allow the student to "keep up" with the flow of patients, recognize the reasons the scan was being performed, and determine what pathologic condition was recognized.

Deborah Lynn Durham, MA, RT(R)(MR)(CT)

ACKNOWLEDGMENTS

I wish to acknowledge all my previous, present, and future students. They lead me to continue researching, exploring, and always trying to make the learning process more effective. I wish to thank Euclid Seeram for all his support and advice during the revision process of this work. Additionally, I extend a special thanks to Julia Casson for all her help and support through e-mails and telephone calls during the past many months. I would also like to extend a special acknowledgment to Dr. Litcher, my professor at Wake Forest University, who helped me with his encouragement during the drafts of this book.

A special thanks always goes to my peers at Forsyth Tech, who listen to me day in and day out, during the good or bad and the fun or serious. They are *always* there for me. You are very, very special. I wish to thank Bill and Carolyn Holland, who took me under their wings 5 years ago and are always there—no matter what! I can never thank you enough for all you do.

—DLD

Patient Care and Safety

Chapter at a glance

Drugs and Outcomes
Radiation Safety and Protection
Computed Tomography Dose Parameters
Factors Affecting Dose
General Statements
Gonadal Shielding
Fetal-Embryonic Effects

INTRODUCTION TO PATIENT CARE AND SAFETY

Patient care in the computed tomography (CT) office must be approached differently compared with the main diagnostic x-ray department. Several factors and topics should be reviewed before starting any CT procedure on any patient. Basic vital signs and other assessment tools must be re-addressed to give the patient the best quality care. Using large amounts of intravenous (IV) and oral contrast in CT sets the stage for potentially dangerous effects on patients depending of course on the known clinical history. Two major complications that occasionally occur include anaphylactic shock and a vasovagal reaction.

The screening process of the patient and the chart lends a clinical history, including allergy recognition and laboratory values for contrast administration or biopsies. Additionally, during the screening process, the patient and family should be educated on the steps involved in a CT scan and why it is necessary for a diagnosis or treatment of a disease process. The patient's physical status should be assessed before and after the CT procedure and any changes should be noted.

SCREENING

The patient should be questioned intensely regarding his or her allergies, cardiac history, and renal history. This data should be as accurate and as up to date as possible. Vital signs should be checked before the CT procedure begins (Table 1-1), which is done routinely at outpatient facilities and occasionally at hospitals. An accurate medical history allows the radiologist and technologist to optimize the procedure to obtain exact information for the referring physician.

TABLE 1-1	Vital Signs		
	BLOOD PRESSURE	RESPIRATIONS	PULSE RATE
Adult	120–140/60–80	10–20/min	65–85 beats/min
Child	120–140/60–80	15–25/min	85–95 beats/min

PULSE LOCALIZATIONS

Pulse count can be achieved by using the following:

- Wrist, carotid, temporal, femoral
- Heart rate
  - ❏ Tachycardia—fast
  - ❏ Bradycardia—slow

INFORMED CONSENT (CONTRAST ADMINISTRATION)

A consent form should always be signed for any invasive procedure having the potential of causing harm to the patient. CT involves the use of contrast and should be explained to the patient for an informed consent to be applicable. The risks of the contrast and the benefits of the procedure should be appropriately defined for the patient in terms he or she can understand. Possible alternative diagnostic testing should be explained as well. Parents or guardians must sign for minors.

PATIENT EDUCATION

An explanation of the CT examination should be provided to every patient. Gaining the patient's confidence will ensure patient cooperation in most circumstances. The equipment can be demonstrated, including rotation of the x-ray tube and movement of the patient couch at specific times during the examination. Noises should be properly noted. Breath-hold instructions are required for spiral scanning. Breathing practice might be of great help to the patient and to the success of the examination. The patient must be made as reasonably comfortable as possible on the patient couch with a pillow underneath the knees. The patient must also have the possible use of contrast explained before the examination for full cooperation to occur. This time is also appropriate for signing the informed-consent form.

PHYSICAL STATUS (HOMEOSTASIS OF THE BODY)

Keeping the body in good equilibrium involves making sure that certain body systems are in good working order. Homeostasis is defined as "equal fluid and electrolyte balance," which depends on all components of the blood that aids in respiration, nutrition, excretion, and protection.

- **Respiration.** Oxygen distribution and carbon dioxide collected for lung expiration
- **Nutrition.** Movement of food, glucose, fats, and acids to body tissues
- **Excretion.** Movement of waste products to excretory system
- **Protection.** Hormone distribution, water balance, and temperature regulation

Several points should be noted regarding the Glasgow Coma Scale (Table 1-2):

- An assessment tool used to note physical status changes
- Based on a scale of 3 to 10, when the number less than 7 can indicate that the patient is in danger
- Assesses three major human responses to different stimuli
  - ❏ Eyes opening
  - ❏ Verbal response
  - ❏ Motor response

ASEPTIC–STERILE TECHNIQUES

Certain techniques involved in the scanning of a patient, such as contrast administration and biopsies, can require aseptic and sterile techniques.

Administrating IV contrast materials via an angiocatheter can have an adverse effect on the patient, whether an allergic

TABLE 1-2		The Glasgow Coma Scale			
EYES OPEN	PTS	VERBAL RESPONSE	PTS	MOTOR RESPONSE	PTS
Spontaneous	4	Oriented	5	Obeys commands	6
Speech	3	Confused speech	4	Localizes pain	5
Pain	2	Inappropriate	3	Withdraws	4
No response	1	Incomprehensible	2	Abnormal flexion	3
		No response	1	Extends	2
				No response	1

reaction to the contrast agent or from using inappropriate techniques and materials for the IV injection.

Aseptic Technique for Intravenous Administration

When performing an invasive procedure, such as the administration of contrast, every effort should be made to create conditions that disallow the presence of pathologic organisms; in other words, a state of sterility. The use of gloves, a Betadine, or an alcohol swab for the injection site is required. All materials (e.g., angiocatheter, tubing, pressure injector parts, contrast) must be checked for contamination before use. The contrast should be specifically checked for foreign particles before loading into the contrast pressure injector.

Assessing Existing Intravenous Administrations

- *Site.* Checked for redness, swelling, and leakage
- *Tubing.* Checked for blood in the line, kinking, and entanglement
- *Bag.* Checked for fluids, hanging securely, and the height of the bag

Site Selection

- No local infiltration or redness should be observed.
- The tourniquet should be placed six to eight inches above the proposed site.
- When inserting the angiocatheter, a 15-degree angle to the vein should be used.
- An angiocatheter is preferred in the CT suite because of the large amounts of contrast used and the ability to withstand the pressure of the automatic injector.

PRESSURE INJECTORS

Pressure injectors are used in the CT scan process to administer the IV contrast in a smooth, consistent way. Injection rates can be set according to the body part that is being imaged.

Equipment

- *Control panel.* Programs the rates, times, and amounts of contrast

- *Heating device.* Keeps loaded contrast at body temperature (directly from the contrast warmer)
- *Syringe.* Removable, disposable, and has different holding capacities

Flow Rate
- Delivery rate per unit of time
- Dependent on viscosity (thickness of fluid), length of tubing, and diameter of tubing

Purpose
- To deliver a consistent flow or bolus of a contrast agent
- To allow good organ perfusion of the contrast
- To increase radiation safety by not requiring personnel to stand in scan room during procedure for manual injection of the contrast

Complications

Generally, complications are not routine when administering IV contrast. The IV does not stay in place for a long period and the amount of fluid is not large. Here is a list of some of the complications that can arise:

- *Infection.* Contamination of the equipment or contrast
- *Infiltration.* IV is out of the vein; swelling and tenderness
- *Embolus.* Air or catheter floating in blood stream; extremely rare
- *Phlebitis.* Streaks up and down the area of injection; area of inflammation

Life-Threatening Situations

Patient assessment and monitoring are crucial in the CT suite because of the invasive nature of the procedure.

- The two most common life-threatening conditions the CT technologist can encounter is anaphylactic shock (contrast) or a vasovagal reaction (trauma or fright).
- A crash cart must be in close proximity to the CT scan room for these emergencies.

Shock

Shock is the interruption of blood flow to vital organs or a lack of the ability of body tissues to use oxygen and nutrients needed.
- Affects all ages
- Caused by injury, disease, or emotional trauma

Symptoms of shock
- Decreased blood pressure
- Weak pulse
- Increased heart rate
- Shallow respiration
- Cyanosis
- Skin pallor
- Restlessness
- Confusion
- Anxiety

Types of shock
- *Hypovolemic.* Loss of blood
- *Septic.* Multiplication of microorganisms in the blood; systemic in nature
- *Cardiogenic.* Inability of heart to pump an adequate blood supply to tissues
- *Neurogenic.* Central nervous system inadequacies
- *Anaphylactic.* Allergic reaction, about which CT technologist is most worried
  - Most common occurrence in CT is reaction to contrast administration.
  - Exaggerated hypersensitivity reaction to antigen previously experienced by the body's immune system.
  - Release of histamines causes vasodilation of vessels and peripheral pooling of blood.
  - Release of histamines also causes contraction of smooth muscles, specifically in the respiratory tract, causing respiratory failure or even death.
  - Symptoms include tightness in chest, itching, urticaria (hives), choking, wheezing, and an increased heart rate.
  - The more sudden the onset is, the more severe the reaction will be.
  - Drug of choice is epinephrine—a bronchodilator (opens bronchioles).

❏ Other drugs given include hydrocortisone, diphenhydramine, and aminophylline

Vasovagal

Vasovagal results from the stimulation of the vagus nerve (10th cranial nerve) causing severe slowing of the heart, which usually causes a sudden loss of consciousness from a decreased cardiac output.

- Can be triggered by pain, fright, or trauma
- Drug of choice: atropine because it increases the heart rate
- The differential symptom between a vasovagal and an anaphylactic reaction is the heart rate

Other Situations
Diabetes

- Disorder of carbohydrate, fat, and protein metabolism, which affects the structure and function of blood vessels
- Causes the pancreas to produce less insulin than necessary or the amount produced does not have the desired effect

Three complications

- *Hypoglycemia.* Insulin reaction; excess amount of insulin in the bloodstream or inadequate food intake to use the insulin. Onset is rapid and action such as ingesting sugar or orange juice must be taken. Hypoglycemia can occur to the CT patient who has been medicated and is then whisked away to the CT department. Symptoms include shaking, nervousness, dizziness, hunger, headache, heavy perspiration, cold, clammy skin, and diminished level of consciousness.
- *Diabetic ketoacidosis.* Insufficient amounts of insulin available to metabolize glucose and to mobilize fatty acids, resulting in an acidotic state. Diabetic ketoacidosis takes longer to develop but is still serious. The patient can be in CT too long and miss an insulin injection. Symptoms include sweet breath odor, warm dry skin, extreme thirst, decreased blood pressure, increased pulse rate, and lethargy.

- *Hyperosmolar coma.* Occurs in older adults and is frequently mistaken as stroke or drunkenness. Hyperosmolar coma is caused by insulin resistance or agents and is life threatening. Patients who are kept NPO (nothing by mouth) are candidates. Symptoms include severe dehydration, dry skin, increased body temperature, thirst, and confusion, ending in a coma state.

INTRAVENOUS CONTRAST AGENTS: CONSIDERATIONS

Two types of IV contrast agents are available: *ionic* and *nonionic*. IV contrast agents are used to highlight any type of tumor, infection, or abnormality in the body. Wherever the contrast travels through the bloodstream and diffuses into abnormal tissue, it causes the area to have a higher absorption of x-rays. Areas of abnormalities visualize as areas of hyperdensity (bright). Dose calculations for the IV contrast should depend on the age and weight of the patient. Most clinical facilities for adult patients use between 100 and 150 ml of an IV contrast agent. With children, the dose calculation in based on 1 ml/pound.

- *Osmolality.* Number of particles per kilogram of solution
- *Osmolarity.* Number of particles per liter of solution

Ionic
- Ratio of iodine to particles in solution (3:2)
- Hyperosmolarity
- More disruptive to the blood brain barrier and the body's systems (more reactions)
- *Osmolality.* 2000 osm/kg

Nonionic
- Ratio of iodine to particles in solution (3:1)
- Hypoosmolarity
- Less disruptive to the blood brain barrier and the body's systems (less reactions)
- *Osmolality.* 600 to 800 osm/kg

Blood
- *Osmolality.* 300 osm/kg

Possible Contraindications to the Use of Intravenous Contrast

Existing disease processes can preclude a patient from receiving an IV contrast agent. All of these agents are filtered through the kidneys and excreted through the urine. Patients with high blood urea nitrogen (BUN) levels and creatinine may not be able to tolerate the contrast. Kidney function would be compromised, thus any disease process that involves the kidneys may prohibit the administration of the IV contrast agent. The following diseases are possible contraindications to the use of IV contrast agents.

- ■ *Pheochromocytoma*
  - ❑ Disease process involving cell tumors of the sympathetic nervous system
  - ❑ Cell tumors produce excessive amounts of catecholamine, epinephrine, and norepinephrine
  - ❑ Patient usually has high blood pressure with a history of diminished urine output
- ■ *Multiple myeloma*
  - ❑ Neoplastic condition that destroys bone
  - ❑ Patient experiences renal dysfunction as a result of convoluted tubules that are blocked by coagulated proteins
- ■ *Sickle cell crisis*
  - ❑ Disease of the blood resulting from a genetic mutation
  - ❑ Erythrocytes have a sickle cell appearance; can cause occlusion of the microcirculation in the body
  - ❑ Renal function is diminished with uremia and decreased urine output
- ■ *Myasthenia gravis*
  - ❑ Neuromuscular disease
  - ❑ Documentation of symptoms exacerbated by IV contrast agents
  - ❑ Respirations affected; can cause respiratory failure

The referring physician and radiologist work together when any of these conditions is present to decide the best alternative or procedure for the diagnosis of the patient's illness.

COMMON LABORATORY VALUES FOR INTRAVENOUS CONTRAST ADMINISTRATION

The ionic and nonionic contrast agents as mentioned are extremely harmful to the kidneys. When this type of contrast agent is needed, certain laboratory values of the patient's blood are checked to make sure their kidneys can manage the load. These laboratory values are as follows:

Creatinine
- Measurement of kidney function
- High value indicates that there is renal impairment, specifically renal glomerulus
- *Gender value differences because of muscle mass*
  - ❏ *Men:* 0.6 to 1.2 mg/dl (milligrams per deciliters)
  - ❏ *Women:* 0.5 to 1.1 mg/dl

Decreased creatinine can be a result of pregnancy, minimal muscle mass, and small stature.

Blood Urea Nitrogen
- Increased BUN is usually associated with kidney disease process.
- Increased BUN can be associated with dehydration.
- Range is 11 to 23 mg/dl.
- Decreased BUN could be a result of liver failure, overhydration, and pregnancy.

COMMON LABORATORY VALUES FOR BIOPSY PROCEDURES

For BUN and creatinine, refer to the values previously detailed. Other laboratory values are also important when preparing for a biopsy. A patient's· bleeding and clotting time must be assessed. These values are obtained by the following tests:

Prothrombin Time
- Measures activity of coagulation in plasma
- Protein produced by liver

- Vitamin K used to manufacture the protein
- Venous blood drawn
- Range is 10 to 14 seconds

Partial Thromboplastin Time
- Substance in the blood that aids in the conversion of other clotting factors
- Time required for clot formation in normal plasma compared with test plasma
- Range is 20 to 35 seconds

Platelets
- Thrombocytes created in blood marrow
- Two thirds in circulatory system
- One third in spleen
- Substance in blood helps with clot formation
- Vascular integrity and vasoconstriction functions
- Used to assess bleeding disorders
- Range is 150 to 450 mm^3

ORAL CONTRAST AGENTS

Oral contrast agents are used to opacify the stomach and bowel for patients undergoing CT scanning. These contrast agents can be administered orally or rectally. Dose calculations again depend on the patient's weight and age. Most clinical facilities administer an average of 1000 ml of oral contrast agents. Contrast agents given rectally usually averages approximately 8 to 10 ml. These contrast agents also cause the tissue to absorb more x-rays, creating an area of hyperdensity. The patient should be screened for allergies to the compounds in the oral contrasts before administering.

- *Water soluble.* Concentration of an iodinated compound is mixed with water.
- *Barium dilution.* 1.5% to 3.0% is needed to opacify the bowel.
  - ❑ *Higher concentrations.* Will cause streaking on the images because of the high x-ray absorption.

Drugs and Outcomes

Refer to Table 1-3 for drugs common to the CT suite.

Radiation Safety and Protection

Understanding the radiation risks involved with CT scanning is important since CT is one of the procedures producing the highest radiation exposure. Additionally, the dose distribution in the patient is different because of the method used to acquire the data. Important facts to remember include:

- Highest radiation exposure examinations occur in CT scanning.
- Manufacturers are required by law to provide a dose table showing doses to patients from their scanner.
- Manufacturers must also provide a radiation scatter distribution chart.
- Physicists use the CT dose parameters discussed below to create these charts.

Computed Tomography Dose Parameters

When discussing the radiation dose in CT, the terms *CT dose index* (CTDI) and *multiple scan average dose* (MSAD) are com-

TABLE 1-3   Drugs Common to the CT Suite

DRUG	ACTION
Chloral hydrate	Sedative
Ativan	Relieves anxiety
Xanax	Relieves anxiety
Dilantin	Seizure control
Percodan	Pain relief
Morphine	Pain relief
Narcan	Reverses respiratory distress
Atropine	Increases heart rate
Dopamine hydrochloride	Increases cardiac output
Epinephrine	Bronchodilator
Heparin	Blood thinner
Versed	Heavy duty sedative

monly used. These terms represent slice dose versus procedure dose. Facts about these terms are as follows:

- CTDI
  - ❏ Ionization chamber used for measurement
  - ❏ Area of dose curve for single slice divided by slice width
- MSAD
  - ❏ Uses CTDI to calculate an average dose in middle of series of CT scans
  - ❏ Ratio of slice width to slice spacing multiplied by CTDI
- The stray radiation dose curve is dumbbell-shaped with the highest radiation in the circle of the gantry (Figure 1-1).
- Technologists should be positioned as far away from patient as possible when in the scan room during data acquisition.

FACTORS AFFECTING DOSE

Several factors influence the dose to the patient. These factors include ones that can and cannot be controlled by the technologist. The equipment and the scan parameters play a major role in dose rates.

- Design of scanner
  - ❏ Scanner type and beam geometry
  - ❏ Collimation system

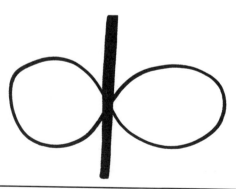

Figure 1-1 Stray radiation dose curve.

- ❑ X-ray spectrum (kilovolt peak [KVP], voltage waveform, tube filtration)
- ❑ Detector
- ■ Controlled factors
  - ❑ Exposure technique factors
  - ❑ Filtration
  - ❑ Collimation
  - ❑ Slice thickness
  - ❑ Slice spacing and the number of adjacent slices
  - ❑ Patient positioning and orientation
  - ❑ Repeat scans
  - ❑ Dynamic versus spiral
  - ❑ Patient characteristics (size, shape, density)

GENERAL STATEMENTS

Some general rules should apply in most CT settings, whether in hospitals or outpatient facilities.

- ■ Walls of CT scan room should be shielded to avoid harm to other personnel and visitors.
- ■ Dose distribution depends on geometry of data gathering and attenuation patterns.
- ■ Dose is greater in the middle of the patient for CT.
- ■ An organ should uniformly absorb radiation.

GONADAL SHIELDING

Shielding should be provided for all patients who are in their childbearing years, women and men. These shielding techniques are somewhat different compared with general radiography.

- ■ Patient must be completely shielded around the body because of the x-ray tube travel.
- ■ Shielding should not cover area of interest or too close so as to cause artifacts.
- ■ Total absorbed dose is smaller in children because of the body volume differences.
- ■ Gonadal exposure comes from internal scatter and not from the beam.
- ■ Shields are now available for patients to protect the eyes, breasts, and thyroid.

FETAL–EMBRYONIC EFFECTS

The first trimester is the most critical stage to avoid radiation because of rapidly developing systems. Radiation to the embryo before implantation usually causes death.

Bioeffects include the following points:

- Absorbed dose is dependent on the type and level of radiation.
- When there is a high rate of energy transfer, more damage will occur.
- Bioeffects depend on the tissue or organ being irradiated.

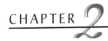

Imaging Procedures

Chapter at a glance

INTRODUCTION TO IMAGING PROCEDURES

Computed tomography (CT) continues to be a complicated technology with evolving techniques. CT uses radiation to obtain axial (transverse) sections through the body. These axial sections can be reformatted into sagittal, coronal, and even oblique sections with the help of specialized postprocessing software. This chapter will examine the definitions of terminology used in the CT scanning process.

ANATOMY AND PHYSIOLOGY

Important anatomic structures that exist throughout the body are used to diagnose certain disease processes. Strategic anatomy for each body system will be discussed. Visualizing the anatomy in the different anatomic planes, either conceptually or by reformatting the CT data, is important. These anatomic planes are (1) sagittal, (2) transverse, (3) coronal, and (4) oblique.

Sagittal Plane
The *sagittal plane* is defined as the plane that passes through the body from right to left or left to right and divides the body into right and left sections.

Transverse Plane
The *transverse plane* is the only plane CT can actually scan in the patient, across the long axis of the body, usually from head to feet or from feet to head (axial).

Coronal Plane
The *coronal plane* is defined as the plane that passes through the body from front to back or back to front, dividing the sections into anterior and posterior slices.

Oblique (Off-Axis) Plane
The *oblique plane* is defined as slanting or deviating from perpendicular or horizontal. An example is paraxial, which is a plane that divides the coronal and sagittal planes in the longitudinal direction of the area.

LANDMARKS

A *landmark* is a physical or visible region of a patient or image that demonstrates the location of specific anatomy. A landmark is also used to set up the scout or to set up a specific transverse slice through a specific region. Landmarks for each of the scanning procedures will be identified appropriately.

CONTRAST MEDIA

The two types of intravenous (IV) contrast agents used are the ionic and nonionic. Both media are usually administered via an automatic pressure injector through a vein in the antecubital area of the arm or on top of the hand. As previously discussed, the pressure injector can be programmed to administer specific amounts of contrast at specific rates (bolus). These amounts and rates are usually site-specific for the type of procedure and disease diagnosis. From 100 to 150 ml of contrast is administered for an adult for a routine CT procedure. For children, the IV contrast agent is administered for a dose of 1.0 milliliter per pound. The purpose of the contrast agent is to highlight abnormalities, tumors, infection, and inflammation in the different body systems. IV contrast is a positive contrast agent in that it absorbs more x-rays and creates a hyperdense area where the abnormality exists. Some structures enhance normally in the body with IV contrast, which will be discussed when appropriate. Four disease processes are known to be possible contraindications for the ionic or nonionic intravenous contrast: multiple myeloma, pheochromocytoma, sickle cell crisis, and myasthenia gravis. (Definitions are presented in Chapter 1.)

The two types of oral contrast are used to opacify the bowel and stomach for the CT scan. Oral contrast helps differentiate fecal material and food from pathological processes. Approximately 1000 ml of the contrast is given by mouth for CT scanning of the abdomen and pelvis. Both the water-soluble and barium dilutions are positive contrast agents because they also absorb more x-rays and create a hyperdense area on the images. Oral contrasts are used for differentiating the bowel and highlighting areas of pathologic conditions.

SCANNING PROCEDURES

Scanning procedures in CT involve the scout scan and the method by which the actual data is acquired using the two most common generation scanners. Comparing conventional and spiral CT acquisitions is also important.

Scout

A patient is positioned on the patient couch. A *scout* or "baby x-ray" is acquired of the area of interest to plot transverse slices of the area under review. A scout can be taken antero-posterior (AP) or lateral (side to side) (Figure 2-1). The x-ray tube and detector array remain stationary for the scout and the patient couch moves through the gantry. Another term for scout is *topogram*.

Data Acquisition

CT scans are acquired transversely with different modes of acquisition depending on the type of scanner and the type of scan being performed.

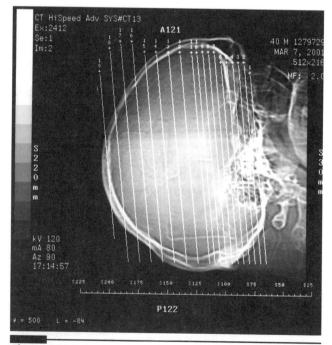

Figure 2-1 Lateral scout of a head.

For third-generation scanners, the x-ray tube and detector array are coupled thus moving together, 360 degrees around patient (Figure 2-2). A ray is defined as an x-ray beam to one detector. A view is defined between angles of the 360-degree sweep around the patient.

For fourth-generation scanners, the x-ray tube moves 360 degrees around the patient. The detectors are stationary in circle of gantry (Figure 2-3). A ray is defined as an x-ray beam to one detector. A view is made up of the rays that hit one detector in a 360-degree sweep. If a particular fourth-generation scanner has 2000 detectors, then each sectional slice will consist of 2000 views.

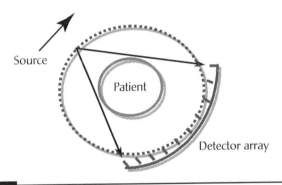

Figure 2-2 Third-generation CT scanner.

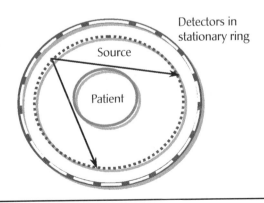

Figure 2-3 Fourth-generation CT scanner.

Conventional. The x-ray tube pulses an x-ray beam as it travels around the patient for data acquisition for a single slice of tissue. The patient couch then moves to the next location for another slice. Conventional scanning can be performed with a spiral or regular CT x-ray tube set-up (cables are attached to the x-ray tube). An interscan delay is required for the patient couch to move, the cabling to unwind, or both.

Spiral-helical scanning. Spiral is defined as the continuous feed of the patient couch into the gantry with continuous rotation of the x-ray tube, similar to a potato peel. A volume of data is acquired during a breath-hold by the patient. Spiral operates with a slip-ring technology in which the x-ray tube travels along concentric rings rather than being attached to cables. Image reconstruction is accomplished by an interpolation algorithm, which synthesizes data from original spiral data.

- ■ Advantages
  - ❏ Complete organ or volume of tissue in one breath-hold
  - ❏ Gapless scanning
  - ❏ Effects of different respirations are removed
  - ❏ Contrast boluses are more effective
  - ❏ More uniform contrast enhancement
  - ❏ Better multiplanar reconstruction and three-dimensional (3-D) imaging
- ■ Disadvantages
  - ❏ Additional demands on the x-ray tube
  - ❏ No defined slice
  - ❏ Effective slice thickness increases because of the influence of a fanned beam and the speed of the table
  - ❏ Projection data is inconsistent

TERMS OF SPIRAL AND HELICAL SCANNING

The CT technologist must be familiar with the terms associated with spiral technology. This level of understanding can affect scanning completeness and patient diagnosis.

- ■ *Pitch.* Distance table travels during one revolution of the x-ray tube.
- ■ *Pitch factor.* Ratio of pitch to the thickness of the slice determines how close the spiral is wound.

- *Image index.* Distance in millimeters between center points of two consecutive reconstructed images; as the index is decreased, the number of images that will be reconstructed is increased.
- *Clinical applications.* Most chest, abdomen, and pelvis CT procedures are scanned using the spiral technique.
  - ❏ *Body.* Chest bolusing, liver lesion detection, and aortic dissection
  - ❏ *3-D.* No gaps in data; no respiratory motion artifacts
  - ❏ *Computerized tomography angiography (CTA).* Volume of data for postprocessing

DYNAMIC COMPUTED TOMOGRAPHY

Dynamic CT is a rapid-scanning method with a short cycle time of scan, reconstruction, and image display. Reconstruction does not necessarily have to occur after each scan, but can occur after a fixed number of slices are acquired. Usually, one slice is acquired repeatedly to watch for contrast flowing in and out of the tissue or organ.

HIGH-RESOLUTION COMPUTED TOMOGRAPHY

High-resolution CT is acquired with a different algorithm, thinner slice thicknesses, and a smaller field of view (FOV) to obtain images with sharper edges of the tissue.

- Frequently performed in the chest to visualize detail of lung markings for interstitial lung diseases
- Slice thicknesses are 1 to 2 mm, taken at specific locations in the chest
- Examples would be at the level of the apices, aortic arch, and the angles of the lung fields
- Algorithm used is bone
- Images appear detailed and sharp
- Used for asbestosis, emphysema, bronchiectasis

PARAMETER SELECTION

A set of x-ray techniques is chosen for the CT scan similar to conventional diagnostic x-ray techniques (Table 2-1). The

TABLE 2-1	Parameter Chart
PARAMETER	DESCRIPTION
kVp	One thousandth of force that will produce a 1 A in circuit with resistance of 1 Ω
mA	One thousandth of an A
mAs	Number of electrons applied to cathode of x-ray tube multiplied by exposure time in seconds; determines amount of x-ray energy produced
Scan FOV	Area scanned by machine
Display FOV	Area of scan FOV to be displayed on monitor
Matrix	Rows and columns of pixels (2-D) representing voxels (3-D volume of tissue) in image
Slice thickness	Thickness of slice
Slice gap	Distance between slices
Algorithm	Mathematic equations (formulas) used to reconstruct data a certain way: *Standard:* For brain, chest, abdomen, pelvis *Detail:* For edge detail (e.g., for neck and face); window widths and window levels are moderate *Bone:* For detail but not contrast resolution (e.g., sinuses, temporal bones, extremity bones); window widths and window levels are widened
Window level	Center of gray scale

FOV, Field of view; *kvp,* kilovolts; *mA,* milliampere; *mAs,* milliamperes per second; *3-D,* three dimensional; *2-D,* two dimensional.

three major algorithms used in CT are the standard, bone, and detail. Each algorithm has its own set of mathematical equations used to create images of different parts of the body.

Recognition of Abnormalities

The CT technologist must recognize an *abnormality* for completeness of the examination and for the proper diagnosis of the patient, as well as recognizing when contrast media or additional scanning is required. Tips for recognizing abnormalities on all types of CT studies include the following:

- Asymmetry from side to side or from anterior to posterior
- Contrast visualization (before and after administering)
- Rough edges around organs

SPECIAL PROCEDURES

Three-Dimensional Studies

- Data acquisition is spiral and thus gapless.
- Common orientations are frontal, top, bottom, rear, left side, and right side to provide a panoramic view.
- Rendering is a process by which CT scan data is converted from a set of slices stored within the CT scanner or workstation into recognizable 3-D images by a computer program.
- Orientation is chosen along with a threshold.
- Thresholds can be low (-150 CT number depicting soft tissue) or high ($+150$ CT number depicting bone).

Surface rendering is a process by which the data are reduced to a set of surfaces on which large scale changes in the threshold occur. This process occurs at boundaries where two different tissue types lie next to each other. Data are extracted and skin is visualized over bone surfaces. Surface rendering is the simplest rendering technique.

Volumetric rendering is a process by which the entire data set is used for generating high-quality, 3-D images. This technique computes from every point in the data set. More computation is required but all information is displayed.

Difficulties. Postprocessing techniques are highly sensitive to motion, thus sedation or anesthesia can be used. Beam hardening artifacts can also occur. Slices in the data set can be lost. Uniform slice thicknesses, magnification factors, and gantry tilt must remain the same for the entire set. Metallic artifacts can be more pronounced and obscure the data set.

Applications. Craniofacial and cardiac work.

Biopsies

CT serves as a useful guide for needle placement into a lesion and helps determine the relationship of the lesion to other structures. CT fluoroscopy is a new popular technique for biopsy precision. Laboratory work to be ordered in case of potential biopsy includes prothrombin time (PT), partial thromboplastin time (PTT), and platelets (see Chapter 1). This laboratory work helps determine blood-clotting viability. Biopsies can be performed anywhere in the body.

Drainage and Aspiration

CT is also used as a guide for tube or line placement into abscesses or areas that must be drained. Again, CT fluoroscopy is available for this procedure.

Radiation Therapy Planning

A board is usually placed on the CT table to mimic the therapy table. The CT is performed in the same position that the therapy will be given. The scan data are sent to the CT computer and then to the radiation therapy computer. Images are used for planning beam positions and depth dose calculations. Isodose curves are plotted and the CT numbers are used to calculate electron densities.

Stereotaxis

Stereotaxis is a method of precisely locating areas of the brain using magnetic resonance or CT guidance. Generally, this procedure is used before neurosurgery and radiation therapy.

CHAPTER 3

Computed Tomography of the Head and Brain

Chapter at a glance

Introduction to Basic Protocols

Head or brain computed tomography (CT) scanning can be performed under routine or emergent conditions. Familiarity with x-sectional anatomy of certain structures and their physiologic significance is important. Basic protocol examples are given for a routine brain and sinus scan. More specific protocol examples are shown for comparison, such as for the temporal bone and orbit (Table 3-1). Common abnormalities of the brain diagnosed with CT will be defined.

Strategic Anatomy

The brain contains numerous subsystems and each is extremely important in every single activity performed during the day by every person. Each subsystem has been divided into smaller and important sections for further reference.

Meninges

- The lining that surrounds and protects the brain.
- *Dura.* Outer layer, which is continuous with the periosteum of the cranium. Between the double layers of dura are the meningeal arteries and the dural sinus tracts.
- *Arachnoid.* Delicate middle layer, which is avascular.
- *Pia.* Inner layer of high vascularity.

Cerebrum

- Largest lobe of the brain; covered by the cerebral cortex
- Gyrus (round lobular structures) and sulcus (grooves between gyrus)
- Two hemispheres (right and left)
- Falx cerebri (dura mater) divider
- Frontal, parietal, temporal, occipital, insula (deepest on internal aspect of hemisphere)
- *Frontal.* Voluntary function, personality
- *Parietal.* Peripheral sensations
- *Temporal.* Smell, taste, hearing
- *Occipital.* Vision
- *Insula.* Motor and sensory function

TABLE 3-1	Routine Protocols for Brain CT
PROTOCOL	DESCRIPTION

Routine head
Standard algorithm

Lateral scout
4–5 mm slices through posterior fossa
7 mm through rest of head
mAs = 340
kVp = 120
Matrix = 256 × 256
DFOV = 220 mm
Usually acquired with and without IV contrast

Sinus
Mini sinus (one slice through each sinus area)
Bone algorithm

Lateral scout
4–5 mm from top of frontal sinus down through end of sphenoid sinus
mAs = 340
kVp = 120
Matrix = 256 × 256, 512 × 512
DFOV = 150 mm
IV contrast dependent

Maxillofacial
Bone algorithm

Lateral scout–anterior to posterior scout
3–4 mm through facial bones
mAs = 340
kVp = 120
Matrix = 256 × 256, 512 = 512
DFOV = 150 mm
IV contrast dependent

Temporal bones
Bone algorithm

Lateral scout–anterior to posterior scout
1–2 mm through petrous ridge (internal auditory canals)
mAs = high because of slice thickness
kVp = 140
Matrix = 512 × 512
DFOV = 150 mm
IV contrast dependent

Orbit
Bone algorithm

Lateral scout
3 mm through orbits axially and coronally; if possible; if not possible, reformats can be done
mAs = up because of slice thickness
kVp = 140
Matrix = 512 × 512
DFOV = 150 mm

DFOV, Display field of view; *IV*, intravenous; *kVp*, kilovolts peak; *mAs*, milliamperes per second.

Cerebellum

- Posterior lobe of brain (Figure 3-1)
- Tentorium separates cerebellum from the cerebrum
- Midline portion (vermis) connects the two cerebellar hemispheres, each having a dentate nucleus; cerebellar tonsils lie on the inferior surface
- Attached to brainstem by three paired bundles of white matter nerve tracts (cerebellar peduncles)
- Location of fourth ventricle
- Coordination for motor skills

Sinus Tracts

- Positioned between visceral and parietal layers of the dura mater
- Venous blood drains into these spaces
- From the sinus tracts into the internal jugular vein:
  - *Superior sagittal.* Triangular shaped; anterior and posterior of axial brain

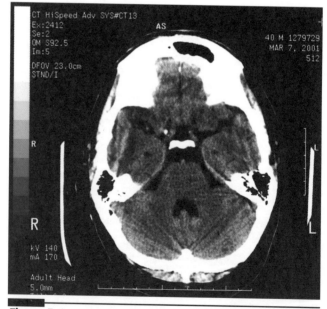

Figure 3-1 CT axial head image shows cerebellum and pons.

❏ *Inferior sagittal.* Inferior margin of falx; ends in straight sinus
❏ *Straight.* Between falx and tentorium
❏ *Transverse.* Laterally to petrous of temporal; in margin of tentorium
❏ *Sigmoid.* Continuation of transverse as it turns inferiorly and medially; becomes the internal jugular vein
❏ *Confluence of sinuses.* Junction of superior sagittal sinus, transverse, straight sinus tracts
❏ *Cavernous.* Either side of sella; communicate with the transverse sinus via the petrosal sinuses

Cisterns

Cisterns are enlarged areas of subarachnoid space filled with cerebrospinal fluid.

- Superior (quadrigeminal)
- Cisterna magnum
- Pontine
- Interpeduncular
- Suprasellar
- Cerebellopontine

Diencephalon

- Part of the forebrain
- Near the third ventricle area, approximately midline
- Epithalamus, thalamus, hypothalamus

White Matter Tracts

- *Corpus callosum.* Genu (anterior), splenium (posterior) midline; largest and densest
- *Internal capsule.* Between caudate nucleus and thalamus and lentiform nucleus
- *External capsule.* Between lentiform nucleus and claustrum
- *Extreme capsule.* Beyond claustrum
- White matter appears hypodense on CT

Basal Ganglia (Gray Matter)

- Collection of subcortical gray matter
- *Caudate nucleus.* Under anterior horns of lateral ventricle

- *Lentiform nucleus.* Globus pallidus and putamen; between internal and external capsules
- *Thalamus.* Positioned on either side of third ventricle
- *Claustrum.* Positioned between external and extreme capsule
- *Gray matter.* Appears hyperdense on CT

Brainstem

- Small mass of tissue connecting the cerebral hemi-spheres with the spinal cord (Figure 3-2)
- *Medulla.* Most inferior section; can visualize vertebral arteries on axial CT; controls heart rate, respirations, and other internal activities; continues as spinal cord
- *Pons.* Middle section, pontine cistern (basilar artery visualized on CT; formed by vertebrals); serves as a bridge between the cerebrum and cerebellum
- *Midbrain.* Observed as heart-shaped or circular-shaped on axial CT scans of brain
  - Tectum is the roof of the midbrain
  - Most superior section; cerebral peduncles-colliculi form top of circle on an axial CT scan
  - Peduncles contain the substantia nigra; produces dopamine
  - Corpora quadrigemina form bottom of circle on scan
  - Cerebral aqueduct can be visualized occasionally in bottom of circle as well

Ventricles

- Produce and provide pathway for cerebrospinal fluid (CSF) (Figure 3-3)
- Lateral ventricles consist of anterior, temporal, posterior horns
- Anterior horns are separated by the septum pellucidum
- Third ventricle lies midline in the axial CT brain
- Fourth ventricle is triangular-shaped; anterior to cere-bellum and posterior to pons
- CSF created in the choroid plexus of the ventricles

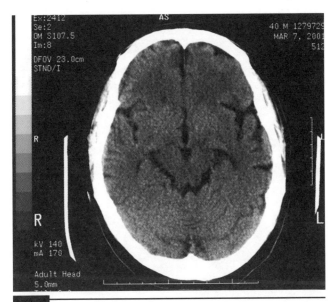

Figure 3-2 CT axial head image showing midbrain section of brainstem.

Flow of Cerebrospinal Fluid
- Lateral ventricles through foramen of Monroe into third ventricle (see Figure 3-3)
- Third ventricle through cerebral aqueduct to fourth ventricle
- Fourth ventricle through foramen of Magendie to spinal canal

Cranial Nerves
- *I–Olfactory.* Smell pathways; neurosensory cells located in nasal conchae
- *II–Optic.* Visual fields; arises from optic retina and goes to posterior aspect of eye
- *III–Oculomotor.* Visual, squinting, ptosis, double vision; supplies nerve fibers to all eye muscles except for the superior oblique and the lateral rectus muscle

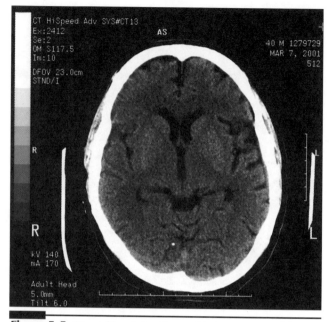

Figure 3-3 CT axial head showing ventricular system and layering of basal ganglia and white matter tracts.

- *IV–Trochlear.* Head tilted to affected side, superior oblique muscle
- *V–Trigeminal.* Largest cranial nerve with three branches (ophthalmic, maxillary, mandibular); pain involvement; major sensory nerve of face; trigeminal neuralgia
- *VI–Abducens.* Eyeball cannot move sideways; directed medially; lateral rectus muscle
- *VII–Facial.* Innervates the facial muscles; provides taste sensation to anterior two thirds of tongue; Bell's palsy
- *VIII–Vestibucochlear.* Vestibular component; aids in equilibrium and cochlear component, which aids in interpretation of sound
- *IX–Glossopharyngeal.* Pain in swallowing; loss of sensation in the throat
- *X–Vagus.* Longest; serves upper body; vasovagal; heart beats, respirations, neck, thorax, abdomen

- *XI–Accessory.* Supplies sternocleidomastoid and trapezius muscle
- *XII–Hypoglossal.* Chewing, swallowing; tongue will curl to affected side; all muscles of tongue except for one

Except for the olfactory and optic nerve, 10 of the 12 cranial nerves arise from the brainstem. In CT, the V, VII, and VIII cranial nerves are of the most concern. Any problems with the V cranial nerve can usually be identified at the cerebellopontine angle, which is the area on either side of the pons. Any abnormality with the VII and VIII cranial nerves can be visualized in the internal auditory canal where these two nerves travel.

Vascular System
- *Circle of Willis*
  - ❏ Anastomosis between four major arteries
  - ❏ Anterior, middle, posterior cerebrals (2)
  - ❏ Anterior communicating (1)
  - ❏ Posterior communicating (2)
  - ❏ Internal carotid arteries
- *Anterior circulation.* Blood to anterior brain supplied via internal carotid artery, which bifurcates into anterior and posterior cerebrals
- *Posterior circulation.* Blood to posterior brain supplied via vertebrales, which form basilar artery, which bifurcates into posterior cerebrals
- *Blood brain barrier*
  - ❏ Endothelial cells lining the capillaries in the central nervous system; controls the chemical exchange between the blood and interstitial fluid
  - ❏ Pressure of a normal blood brain barrier prevents large amounts of contrast medium from entering the brain

Ear
- *Inner ear*
  - ❏ Fluid-filled containing vestibule, semicircular canals, cochlea
  - ❏ Equilibrium, balance, hearing
  - ❏ Communication with middle ear through oval window

- *Middle ear*
  - ❑ Air-filled tympanic cavity
  - ❑ Tympanic membrane and three ossicles (malleus, incus, stapes)
  - ❑ Connects with pharynx through eustachian tube for pressure equalization
- *External ear*
  - ❑ Auricle and external auditory meatus and external auditory canal
  - ❑ Auricle directs sounds into auditory canal ending at tympanic membrane

Orbit

- *Bony.* Junction of frontal, sphenoid, ethmoid bones of cranium and lacrimal, palatine, maxillary, zygomatic bones of face
- *Eye*
  - ❑ Anterior compartment in front of lens containing cornea and iris; filled with aqueous humor
  - ❑ Posterior compartment surrounded by retina contains vitreous humor
- *Muscles*
  - ❑ Medial, lateral, superior, inferior rectus
  - ❑ Superior and inferior oblique; act to abduct, adduct, rotate eyeball
- *Optic nerve*
  - ❑ Between medial and lateral rectus on CT axial scan
  - ❑ Lies in retroorbital fat
  - ❑ Carries information from retina to optic chiasm, to thalamus gland, to visual cortex of cerebral hemisphere

Bony Cranium

- *Occipital.* Forms posterior cranial fossa
- *Temporal.* Creates the middle cranial fossa
- *Sphenoid.* Extends across floor of middle cranial fossa; butterfly shaped
- *Ethmoid.* Positioned in anterior cranial fossa
- *Frontal.* Anterior vault of cranium
- *Parietal.* Sides of cranium

Facial Bones

- *Six paired bones.* Inferior nasal conchae, lacrimal, maxilla, palatine, zygomatic
- *Two unpaired bones.* Vomer, mandible
- *Major muscles.* Temporalis, buccinator, masseter; help with movement of jaws and face

Glands

- *Pituitary*
  - ❏ Endocrine gland located in sella turcica
  - ❏ Master gland producing numerous hormones relating to growth, reproduction, various metabolic activities
  - ❏ Anterior and posterior lobes
- *Pineal*
  - ❏ Pine cone-shaped; located dorsal to third ventricle
  - ❏ Superior to midbrain
  - ❏ Secretes melatonin; hormone responsible for regulating biologic rhythms; promotes sleep

SPECIFIC PROTOCOLS

Several specific structures in the brain require their own special protocol or set of parameters. These structures include the sella, sinuses, and temporal bones. Routine brain imaging will be reviewed. (For specific parameter protocols, see Table 3-1.)

Sella

The pituitary gland, positioned in the sella turcica, is usually imaged by magnetic resonance imaging (MRI). When scanned in CT, reconstructions in the sagittal and coronal plane are required. Thinner cuts and contrast are necessary. A lateral scout is acquired to set up the scan slices. The pituitary gland takes up the contrast quickly, thus a tumor would appear hypodense on the scan. After the gland has washed out the contrast, the tumor will eventually enhance and appear hyperdense.

Sinus

To best visualize air fluid levels in the sinuses, the patient should be positioned prone with the head and neck extended.

Data acquisition in this position creates direct coronals. Thinner cuts should be used (see Table 3-1). A lateral scout is performed to set up the scan slices.

Temporal Bones

Temporal bones are scanned to visualize the ear. Thinner cuts (1 to 2 mm) should be acquired with or without contrast. A lateral and an anterior to posterior scouts are acquired to fully visualize the petrous ridge to set up appropriate scan levels.

Routine

Scans acquired before and after administrating a contrast agent are performed for a routine CT of the head. Usually, 5 mm slice thicknesses are acquired through the posterior fossa (cerebellum), then 8 mm slice thicknesses throughout the rest of the brain. A lateral scout is acquired to set up the scans at the appropriate angle.

COMMON ABNORMALITIES OF THE BRAIN

Several abnormalities can be diagnosed with CT. Different types of tumors, infections, and hemorrhages have been well documented using the CT imaging modality.

Intraaxial Tumors of the Brain

- Arise from the brain tissue itself
- Examples include:
    - *Gliomas.* Aggressive malignant tumors; different categories; majority of thalamic tumors
    - *Metastasis.* Cells from a primary cancer grow into tumors at the gray-white matter junctions of the brain tissue
    - *Tumors.* Mixed density pattern with leaflike or irregular projections into white matter
- *Frontal lobe tumors.* Seizures, behavioral and personality changes, dementia
- *Parietal lobe tumors.* Aphasia; right or left contusions
- *Temporal lobe tumors.* Seizures, psychomotor, aphasia
- *Occipital lobe tumors.* Hemianopsia, visual field defects, focal vision problems

- *Corpus callosum lesions.* Increased intracranial pressure, personality-behavioral changes, seizures, alexia (inability to read)
- *Lateral ventricle lesions.* Hydrocephalus with ventricular obstruction
- *Basal ganglia lesions.* Progressive worsening of motor and sensory disturbances, Parkinson's disease
- *Thalamus lesions.* Lateral extension of tumor causes hemiparesis and hemisensory deficits; posterior extension causes impaired ventricle movements, pupil abnormality, hemianopsia
- *Tentorial lesions.* Trigeminal neuralgia-facial pain, gait instability, cranial nerve palsies
- *Brain stem lesions.* Cranial nerve paresis; vomiting or nausea; gait disturbances
- *Cerebellar lesions.* Intracranial hypertension without clear-out signs; unilateral limb ataxia; balance; gait abnormalities

Extraaxial Tumors of the Brain

- Arise from outside of the brain tissue
- Examples include:
  - *Acoustic neuroma.* Tumors occurring on the eighth cranial nerve, which courses through the internal auditory canal
  - *Meningioma.* Encapsulated benign tumor appearing isodense on CT scans, but enhances uniformly with the IV contrast; regular in shape and sharply marginated

Hemorrhages

- *Subdural.* Collection of venous blood between the dura and subarachnoid space as a result of the rupture of bridging veins, which connect to venous sinuses, usually a result of trauma; blood appears white on CT scans of the brain; do not cross midline
- *Epidural.* Collection of arterial blood in the epidural space as a result of a rupture of the meningeal artery, usually a result of trauma; extremely serious condition because of arterial blood loss; blood appears white on CT scans of the brain; can cross midline

■ *Subarachnoid.* Collection of blood in the space between the arachnoid and pia mater, usually caused by rupture of a Berry aneurysm at a bifurcation in the Circle of Willis in the brain; can be caused by a leak or rupture in an arteriovenous malformation (tangle of abnormal vessels with varying diameters–large feeding arteries and large draining veins–occurring in cerebral hemispheres); blood appears white on CT scans of the brain

■ *Intercerebral.* Blood from a hemorrhagic stroke or trauma; can occur anywhere in the brain; blood appears white on CT scans of the brain

Other Disease Processes

■ *Hydrocephalus.* Increased cerebrospinal fluid in the ventricles in the brain, caused by either a blockage or tumor in the system or a congenital abnormality; enlarged ventricles could cause pressure on other brain tissue

■ *Stroke.* An area of ischemia in the brain from cut off circulation; tissue will die; dead tissue will attenuate the x-ray beam differently; strokes do not visualize on CT scans until after 48 to 72 hours have passed; shown as a hypodense area on the scan. Strokes can appear as fan-shaped or triangular-shaped and conform to specific vascular territories. Table 3-2 shows how a stroke would visualize on CT, depending on how old the stroke is.

TABLE 3-2 **Stroke: Age versus Appearance**

AGE OF STROKE	CT APPEARANCE
Immediate	None
Hyperacute (less than 12 hrs)	Normal (50%–60%)
	Hyperdense artery (25%–50%)
Acute (12–24 hrs)	Loss of gray-white interfaces
	Sulcal effacement
	Low density of basal ganglia
1–3 days	Mass effect
	Wedge-shaped, low-density area
4–7 days	Hemorrhagic transformation
	Gyral enhancement
1–8 wks	Mass effect and edema persist
	Contrast enhancement persists
	Mass effect resolves
Months–years	Volume loss
	Encephalomalacic change

- ■ *Abscess.* Circumscribed collection of pus occurring in an acute or chronic infection in the brain tissue; with administration of contrast, abscess will show ring enhancement
- ■ *Pituitary tumor.* Mass arising from posterior or anterior lobe of gland; microadenoma is less than 1 cm; macro-adenoma is more than 1 cm
- ■ *Encephalitis.* Inflammation of the brain tissue
- ■ *Meningitis.* Inflammation of the meninges
- ■ *Cholesteatoma.* Squamous epithelium forms a pearly white mass from chronic and acute inflammations in the middle ear

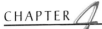
Computed Tomography of the Neck

Chapter at a glance

INTRODUCTION TO BASIC PROTOCOLS

Computed tomography (CT) scanning of the soft tissue of the neck uses a smaller field of view (FOV) compared with head scanning. Slice thicknesses depend on structures to be imaged. Soft tissue neck protocols are written to look specifically at some of the smaller structures of the neck, such as the salivary glands, larynx, or pharynx (Table 4-1). Important anatomy to be visualized will be defined, as well as common diseases involving the soft tissue neck.

TABLE 4-1	Soft Tissue Neck Protocols
PROTOCOL	DESCRIPTION
Nasopharynx	Lateral scout 3–10 mm slice thickness Detail algorithm Contrast for tumor enhancement Scan from hard palate to temporal bone Can acquire direct coronals with patient prone
Larynx	Lateral scout No swallowing Detail algorithm Small FOV Phonation of the letter e to check vocal cord mobility 3 mm slice thickness angled to plane of vocal cords (usually angle of cervical disk spaces) Scan from base of tongue to crinoid cartilage
Parotid gland	Lateral scout 3–6 mm slice thickness High-resolution algorithm Small FOV Angle scans to avoid dental fillings Contrast for tumor enhancement Scan from zygomatic arches to below mandibular angle
Submandibular gland	Scan from mandibular angle to hyoid bone
Cancer of the throat	Lateral scout 3–5 mm slice thickness Detail algorithm

FOV, Field of view.

The neck can be positioned straight or hyperextended to some degree. This positioning depends on what the focus of the procedure is (i.e., the area of interest).

STRATEGIC ANATOMY

Specific structures in the neck must be visualized to complete an examination. Generally, an invasion of a lesion into the glands or into the vascular components of the neck is being diagnosed. These structures will now be examined.

Salivary Glands

- *Parotid.* High fatty content allows good visualization on the CT scan
  - *Location.* On the posterior border of the mandible between the ramus of the mandible and the sternocleidomastoid muscle
  - *Size.* Largest of the salivary glands
- *Submandibular.* Lies internal to the body of the mandible
- *Sublingual.* Lies underneath the tongue; smallest of the salivary glands

Pharynx

- Long, funnel-shaped muscular tube from base of skull downward until it eventually becomes the esophagus
- Acts as opening for respiration and digestive tracts
  - *Nasopharynx.* Behind the nose; superior to trachea
  - *Oropharynx.* Behind the mouth; soft palate to hyoid bone
  - *Laryngopharynx.* Behind the larynx; oropharynx to esophagus
  - *Retropharyngeal space.* Space behind the pharynx; reviewed for extension of disease processes

Larynx

- Beginning of respiration pathway
- Reinforced by cartilage
- Location of true-false vocal cords

Trachea

- Reinforced by C-shaped cartilage
- Tube down into lungs, becomes the right and left main stem bronchus; sits anterior to the pharynx (esophagus); common carotid arteries sit on either side, as does the thyroid gland (endocrine gland)

Thyroid Glands

- Two lobes on either side of trachea
- Hormones produced govern metabolic rate of body

Parathyroid Glands
- Lie on posterior surface of thyroid
- Secrete hormone that monitors concentration of calcium ions in body fluids

Esophagus
- Continuation of pharynx; becomes digestive tract into stomach
- Sits posterior to trachea on an axial CT scan through the area

Vascular Components
- *Internal jugulars.* The right internal jugular is larger than the left; drains into the subclavian vein, which drains into the brachiocephalic vein, then superior vena cava
- *External jugulars.* Sit laterally near the sternocleidomastoid muscle, near the parotid gland
- *Common carotids.* Branch into internal and external at C-5 (internal supplies the brain; external supplies the face); right common carotid is a branch of the brachiocephalic artery; left common carotid is a branch of the aortic arch; external carotid sits anterior to the internal carotid
- *Vertebrals.* Branch of the subclavian artery; these course through the transverse foramina of the cervical vertebrae, up the spinal column, until the two join to form the basilar at approximately the level of the pons (brainstem)
- *Carotid sheath.* Compartment composed of cervical fascia enclosing the common and internal carotid arteries, internal jugular veins, lymph nodes, vagus nerve

Muscles
- *Facial expression*
  - *Temporalis.* Appears with the zygomatic arch
  - *Masseter.* Lateral to the ramus of the mandible
  - *Pterygoid.* Medial to the ramus of the mandible
- *Neck muscles*
  - *Sternocleidomastoid muscle.* Posterior to the parotid gland; sits in the lateral neck; straplike muscle used to turn the head from side to side

❑ *Trapezius muscles.* Sits more posterior in the neck; posterior portion of neck to elevate the scapula
❑ Both are served by the accessory (II) cranial nerve
❑ *Platysma.* Anterior surface of the neck

Lymph Nodes

Chains of lymph nodes are clustered in the neck around the vascular and muscular structure.

Nerves

■ *Vagus nerve (X).* Travels down through the neck; longest cranial nerve
■ *Cervical plexus.* Also lies in the neck area; a network of nerve fibers serving the arms; involves spinal nerve pairs C-1 through C-8; part of the plexus is the extremely important phrenic nerve, which controls diaphragm movement

COMMON ABNORMALITIES OF THE NECK

Common abnormalities of the neck include a variety of tumors of the parotid, cancers of the neck, and thyroid disease.

Parotid Cyst or Lesion

Fluid-filled cysts in the parotid gland could be components of a more serious lesion. Parotid lesions are usually biopsied.

Neck Cancer

Cancers in the neck can be of different types. Lymphoma is nodular or ulcerative in nature. Squamous cell carcinoma is when squamous cells grow abnormally and progress to an ulcerative nature.

Other Disease Processes

■ *Hyperthyroidism.* Increases in heart rate, blood pressure level, metabolic rate
■ *Hypothyroidism.* Decreases in metabolic rate, lethargy, slowed reflexes
■ *Goiter.* Enlargement of the thyroid gland; inability of the gland to synthesize and release adequate amounts of the thyroid hormone

CHAPTER 5

Computed Tomography of the Spine

Chapter at a glance

INTRODUCTION TO BASIC PROTOCOLS

The spinal column consists of 33 vertebrae, separated into cervical, thoracic, lumbar, sacral, and coccyx regions. Computed tomography (CT) of the spine can be performed with or without thecal sac dye from a myelogram, and they can be scanned with or without intravenous (IV) contrast. Both of these procedures depend on the history and probable diagnosis of the patient. Protocols for the cervical, thoracic, and lumbar spine are similar (Table 5-1). In essence, the difference among these protocols lies in the field of view (FOV) and slice thickness.

Strategic Anatomy

When diagnosing a spinal disease, different parts of the spine and different structures in each part should be examined. The bones, muscles, ligaments, and nerves must be identified for certain procedures.

Cervical Spine

- Seven vertebrae; one = atlas, two = axis
- Transverse foramina through which vertebral arteries travel
- Bifid spinous processes, except for C7

Thoracic Spine

- 12 vertebrae
- Facets on transverse processes for rib articulations; costotransverse joints
- Articulations between ribs and vertebral bodies; costovertebral joints
- Long and slender spinous processes, which project inferiorly over vertebral arches

Table 5-1	**Examples of Spine Protocols**
PROTOCOL	DESCRIPTIONS
Spine (standard)	Lateral scout
	3–4 mm angled through disk spaces
	mAs = 550
	kVp = 120
	Matrix = 256 × 256, 512 × 512
	DFOV = 180
	IV contrast dependent
	Spines sometimes done after myelography with contrast in the thecal sac

DFOV, Detailed field of view; *IV*, intravenous; *kVp*, kilovolts peak; *mAs*, milliamperes per second.

Lumbar Spine
- Five vertebrae
- Support posterior abdominal wall
- Large massive bodies with short spinous processes; the largest is L5
- Spinal cord ends at approximately L2 with the meninges, subarachnoid space; cerebrospinal fluid continuing to S2

Sacrum
- Five fused vertebrae
- Transverse processes (lateral masses or ala)
- Sacral foramina for nerve pathways

Coccyx
- Tailbone; posterior projections
- Three to five small fused bones

Parts of the Vertebra
- Vertebral body (Figure 5-1)
- Lamina
- Pedicle
- Superior articular process and inferior articular process, which make up the apophyseal joint

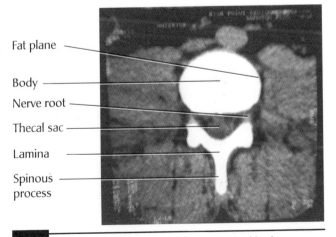

Fat plane

Body

Nerve root

Thecal sac

Lamina

Spinous
process

Figure 5-1 CT axial lumbar spine shows vertebral body.

- Epidural fat, which surrounds the spinal meninges
- Nerve roots (dorsal and ventral)
- *Ligamentum flavum.* Yellow ligament, which joins the lamina of adjacent vertebral arches

Terminology and Structures

- *Nucleus pulposus.* Soft gelatinous disk material (Figure 5-2)
- *Annulus fibrosis.* Cartilaginous outer lining around disk material
- *Spinal cord*
  - ❏ Made up of white and gray matter; white matter surrounds gray matter
  - ❏ Amount of gray matters gets smaller as scan moves from cervical to lumbar region
  - ❏ Surrounded by spinal meninges
- *Conus medullaris.* Tapering end of spinal cord ending at L1 or L2
- *Cauda equina.* Nerve endings tapering the rest of the spinal or thecal sac, eventually attaching to coccyx
- *Spinal nerves*
  - ❏ 31 pairs
  - ❏ Ventral and dorsal nerve roots unite to form the pair

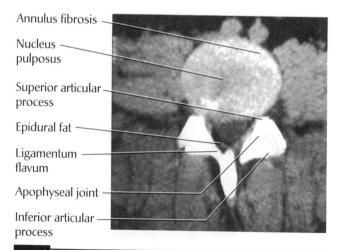

Annulus fibrosis

Nucleus pulposus

Superior articular process

Epidural fat

Ligamentum flavum

Apophyseal joint

Inferior articular process

Figure 5-2 CT axial spine shows soft tissue disk material.

- *Nerve roots*
  - ❏ *Ventral-efferent.* Motor functions
  - ❏ *Dorsal-afferent.* Sensory functions

Muscles
- *Superficial group*
  - ❏ Trapezius and latissimus dorsi help with movement of upper limbs
  - ❏ Serratus posterior helps in respiration movement
- *Erector spinae group*
  - ❏ Massive muscles create prominent bulge on each side of the vertebral column
  - ❏ Three vertical columns of the iliocostalis, longissimus, spinalis
  - ❏ Chief extensors of the spine
- *Transversospinal group*
  - ❏ Deepest layer along the grooves of the spinous and transverse process
  - ❏ Multifidus is the largest
  - ❏ The psoas lies along the lateral aspect of the lumbar spine

Plexuses
- Ventral rami of all spinal nerves, except for T2 through T12
- Networks of nerves and fibers to either side of the body
- *Cervical*
  - ❏ Phrenic nerve (diaphragm)
  - ❏ Ventral rami of C1 through C8
  - ❏ Muscles of shoulder and neck
- *Brachial*
  - ❏ C5 through C8 and T1
  - ❏ Middle and anterior scalene muscles to axilla
- *Lumbar*
  - ❏ T12, L1 through L4, S1 through S4
  - ❏ Lower abdominopelvic region, buttocks, anterior thighs
- *Sacral*
  - ❏ Sciatic nerve
  - ❏ L4 and L5 and S1 through S4
  - ❏ Lower trunk and posterior thighs and feet

Spinal Vasculature

- **Spinal arteries**
    - ❑ Travel with the spinal nerves; divide into dorsal and ventral arteries
    - ❑ Formed channels that divide into a single anterior spinal artery and a pair of posterior spinal arteries
    - ❑ Vertebral and segmental arteries along the spinal cord
- **Spinal veins**
    - ❑ Internal and external plexuses communicate with venous sinuses of the brain
    - ❑ Plexuses drain the basivertebral veins, which drain the vertebral bodies

Specific Protocols

Filming

Spine CT images are filmed or windowed in two different ways. One way visualizes the soft tissue disk material and the other visualizes the bones of the spine. The scans can be angled to the intervertebral disk space or they can be straight with no angle. Some spine CT scans are performed after the patient has undergone a myelogram. Postmyelogram CT spine procedures are performed within 4 to 6 hours after the myelogram. The patient is rolled before the scan to ensure that the contrast in the thecal sac is appropriately mixed again. Postmyelogram CTs are scanned with an angle to the intervertebral disk space thus showing lateral disk herniations better.

Postmyelography

With cervical CT scans, the FOV is smaller. A 3 mm slice thickness is used with an overlap. A standard or bone algorithm is also used. With thoracic and lumbar CT scans, the slice thickness used is 4 to 5 mm with an overlap. CT scans of the spine look for scar tissue after spinal surgery, infections, or tumors.

Common Abnormalities of the Spine

Several conditions of the spine can be diagnosed with CT, including tumors, infections, congenital abnormalities, and fractures.

Tumor Classifications

- **Extradural tumors**
  - ❏ Arise from bones or from the dural space
  - ❏ 90% are malignant; usually metastasis from breast or lung cancer
- **Intradural tumors.** Within dural space (intramedullary and extramedullary)
  - ❏ *Intramedullary tumors*
    - Arise from within the spinal cord itself
    - Grow in central part of spinal cord; destroy fibers and creating a syrinx (fluid-filled cavity)
    - Gliomas are an example, which are not as aggressive as in the brain tissue
  - ❏ *Extramedullary tumors*
    - Arise in between the dura and spinal cord
    - Meningiomas are examples, 90% of which are in the thoracic region
    - Neurofibromas are another example, which arise from the dorsal nerve root
- Most tumor diagnosis is now accomplished with magnetic resonance imaging (MRI).

Disk Herniation

- A tear in the annulus fibrosis through which the nucleus pulposus is protruding
  - ❏ Against the thecal sac (ventrally)
  - ❏ Against the nerve root (posterolaterally)
  - ❏ Common at L4 and L5 or L5 and S1
  - ❏ Common at C5 and C6
- **Bulging disk.** Annulus fibrosus remains intact while disk expands in a symmetrical fashion

Occasionally, a contrast agent is used to enhance the epidural veins and mark the boundaries of the disk material.

Spinal Stenosis

Spinal stenosis is a reduction of available space in the spinal column causing compression of the neural elements. This condition fosters the growth of osteophytes and the degeneration process.

Spondylosis

Spondylosis is characterized by the immobility and consolidation of the joints between the vertebral bodies.

Spondylolisthesis

Spondylolisthesis is characterized by the anterior displacement or slipping of vertebrae, usually at L4 and L5 and at L5 and S1.

Vacuum Phenomenon

Vacuum phenomenon is characterized by nitrogen gas forming in the nucleus pulposus as a result of a degenerative disease.

Fractures

- Scans performed for reformatting of images looking for displaced fragments
- Bony encroachment on the spinal cord
  - *Chance fracture.* "Seat Belt"; usually at L1 or L2; consists of a horizontal fracture through all portions of vertebrae and is usually stable
  - *Clay-shoveler fracture.* Avulsion fracture of C7; first reported in individuals with fractures caused by shoveling wet clay
  - *Hangman fracture.* Bilateral fracture through the pedicles or dislocation of C2; usually caused by a hyperextension type injury; considered unstable
  - *Jefferson fracture.* Compression-type injury to the anterior and posterior arches of C1, resulting in the displacement of the lateral masses; known as a *diving injury*
  - *Odontoid fracture.*
    - 1: Fracture in the upper part of the odontoid; stable and rare
    - 2: Fracture in the base of the odontoid; unstable
    - 3: Fracture through the base of odontoid into the body of C-1; stable
  - *Teardrop fracture.* Spinal fracture resulting in teardrop segment avulsed from part of body or spinous process; unstable and dangerous when close to spinal cord

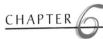
Computed Tomography of the Chest

Chapter at a glance

INTRODUCTION TO BASIC PROTOCOLS

Computed tomography (CT) scans of the chest are performed with the spiral breath-hold technique. Parameters used for chest imaging are included in Table 6-1. Intravenous (IV) contrast is routinely used for chest imaging to differentiate vessels from mediastinal structures. Spiral allows fast imaging to obtain visualization of the great vessels in the mediastinum. The mediastinum, great vessels, heart, and lung fields are main structures for visualization in chest imaging.

STRATEGIC ANATOMY

The chest area contains several different kinds of important anatomy ranging from bony components to the heart. Other important structures are the great vessels and the lung fields. Each one of these components is important for patient diagnosis.

TABLE 6-1	Chest Protocols
PROTOCOL	DESCRIPTION
Routine chest (standard) Spiral (breath-hold)	Anterior to posterior scout (7 mm from top of apex of lungs down through the liver and adrenal glands if questionable cancer staging) mAs = 275 kVp = 130 Matrix = 256 × 256 DFOV = 400 mm IV contrast with pressure injector usage

DFOV, Display field of view; *IV,* intravenous; *kVp,* kilovolts peak; *mAs,* milli-amperes per second.

Bony Components

- Thoracic vertebrae (12)
- Sternum (manubrium, body, xiphoid)
- Ribs with costal cartilage attachments
- *Jugular notch.* Superior border of the manubrium (top of sternum): a common landmark
- *Sternal angle.* T4 and T5, where the manubrium and body of the sternum combine to form a ridge, another common landmark

Thoracic Components

- *Inlet.* Superior aperture for passage of nerves, vessels, and viscera from neck to chest
- *Outlet.* Inferior aperture for passage of nerves, vessels, and visceral from chest to abdomen

Lung Tissue

- Upper field is apex
- Apex to diaphragm
- *Pleural cavity.* Serous membrane lines this cavity; divided into parietal and visceral layers
- *Cardiac notch.* Large notch on medial surface of left lung
- *Hilum.* Passage for main stem bronchi, blood, lymph, nerves to enter the lung
- *Trachea.* Branches into the right and left stem bronchi; occurs at the carina at T-5; bronchial tree divides until becoming alveoli, which are the units of respiration

Mediastinal Area

- Area of soft tissue structures between the lungs
- *Thymus gland.* Posterior to the manubrium and becomes smaller as aging takes place; a role in development of immune system
- *Trachea.* Anterior to the esophagus in the axial CT chest until the trachea bifurcates into the bronchi and the esophagus; drains into the stomach
- *Thyroid gland.* On either side of the trachea in upper axial CT chest scans
- *Great vessels.* Aortic arch, descending aorta, superior vena cava; all are in the mediastinum
- *Thoracic duct.* The main vessel of the lymph system; ascends thorax lying between the azygos vein and descending aorta
- *Lymph nodes.* Also a part of the mediastinum

Diaphragm

- *Chief muscle of inspiration.* Spans entire thoracic outlet; attaches to lumbar spine via the crura
- *Crura of the diaphragm.* Extend inferiorly, nearly past the liver
- *Aortic hiatus.* Opening in diaphragm through which the descending aorta, azygos vein, and thoracic duct pass
- *Cardiac hiatus.* Opening through which the inferior vena cava and the right phrenic nerve pass
- *Esophageal hiatus.* Opening through which the esophagus and the vagus nerve pass

Muscles

- *Pectoralis major and minor.* Anterior surface of chest; movement of the upper limbs
- *Serratus anterior and posterior.* Form parenthesis around lung fields; holds scapula against thorax
- *Rhomboid.* Muscle deep to the trapezius
- *Trapezius.* Posterior around shoulder area
- *Scalene.* Around which brachial plexus is located
- *Intercostal.* Three layers; elevate ribs

Vasculature

- Upper chest vessels (Figure 6-1)
- *Carotids and subclavian arteries.* On either side of the trachea and esophagus, which sit midline
- *Brachiocephalic veins.* Below the clavicles (external jugular into subclavian veins, which become these veins)
- *Aortic arch* (Figure 6-2)
  - ❑ *First branch.* Brachiocephalic, which branches into right common carotid and right subclavian
  - ❑ *Second branch.* Left common carotid
  - ❑ *Third branch.* Left subclavian
- *Superior vena cava.* Formed from brachiocephalic veins (left comes over the brachiocephalic artery and joins the right to become the superior vena cava)
- *Pulmonary trunk.* Scanning from superior to inferior in the chest, the left pulmonary artery is seen first before the pulmonary trunk from which it branches (Figure 6-3). Four pulmonary veins enter the left atrium from the lungs.
- *Azygos venous*
  - ❑ Collateral circulation between inferior vena cava and superior vena cava

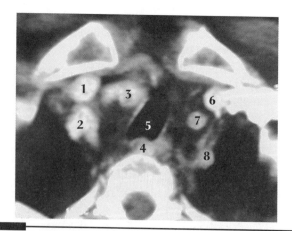

Figure 6-1 Axial chest CT shows upper chest vessels. *1,* Right brachiocephalic vein; *2,* right subclavian artery; *3,* right common carotid; *4,* esophagus; *5,* trachea; *6,* left brachiocephalic vein; *7,* left common carotid artery; *8,* left subclavian artery.

- ❑ Azygos and hemiazygos
- ❑ Azygos sits on the right side of the vertebral column; drains into the superior vena cava

Heart

- ■ *Four chambers.* Left atrium, right atrium, right ventricle, left ventricle (Figure 6-4)
- ■ *Atria.* Superior collecting chambers

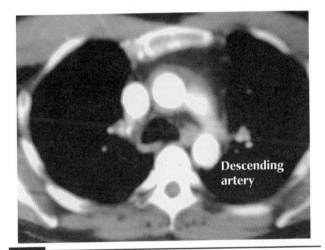

Figure 6-2 Axial chest CT identifying arch splitting into ascending and descending aorta.

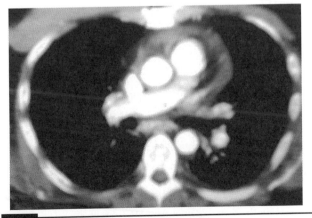

Figure 6-3 Axial chest CT depicts pulmonary trunk.

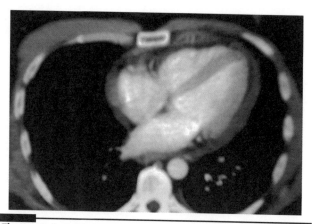

Figure 6-4 Axial chest CT through the chambers of the heart.

- ■ *Ventricles.* Inferior pumping chambers
- ■ *Interarterial septum.* Divides the atria
- ■ *Interventricular septum.* Divides the ventricles
- ■ *Valves.* One-way flow
- ■ *Coronary arteries.* Supply blood supply to the heart muscle
- ■ *Pericardium.* Lining around the heart
- ■ *Apex.* Most inferior part of the heart
- ■ *Base.* Most superior part of the heart
- ■ *Epicardial fat.* Lies between the pericardium and the heart wall
- ■ *Walls.* Three layers—epicardium, myocardium, endocardium
- ■ *Box method.* Identifies chambers of the heart

SPECIFIC PROTOCOLS

Contrast is routinely used for chest CT. With the importance of contrast bolusing in the chest to diagnose different diseases, the use of spiral CT is necessary. The spiral CT is the continuous movement of the patient couch into the gantry during continuous rotation of the x-ray tube, which provides a volume of data compared with slice-by-slice CT. Better differentiation between vessels and mediastinal structures such as lymph nodes can be accomplished with contrast in the great vessels. Routine rates are included in Table 6-2. A CT scan of the chest

TABLE 6-2	**Power Injector Parameters for Chest Imaging**
ROUTINE DELAY TIMES FOR CONTRASTING THE CHEST	
Flow rate: 2.0–2.5 cc/sec (150 cc total contrast)	10 second delay before scan start

through the liver and adrenal glands can be accomplished in one breath-hold of the patient. The adrenal glands are the first place for a lung cancer to metastasize.

Chest CT scans are routinely filmed two different ways. One way visualizes the soft tissue and vessels in the mediastinum. The other way visualizes the feathery markings of the lung tissue.

HIGH-RESOLUTION COMPUTED TOMOGRAPHY OF THE CHEST

High-resolution CT is used mostly in chest imaging. Listed are important facts regarding high-resolution CT imaging and instances for which it would be used.

- Can use smaller detailed field of view (DFOV)
- 1 to 2 mm slice thicknesses at predesignated locations in the chest
- Bone algorithm is used to show feathery lung markings
- Used for interstitial lung diseases (emphysema, asbestos, bronchiectasis)
  - *Emphysema.* Abnormally expanded or destroyed air spaces distal to terminal bronchioles
  - *Asbestosis.* Chest disease from inhaling asbestos; interstitial lung damage
  - *Bronchiectasis.* Irreversible dilation of the bronchi; most common in lower lobes; bilateral

COMMON ABNORMALITIES OF THE CHEST

Abnormalities of the chest can be placed into two sections: respiratory and cardiovascular. The chest is composed mostly of lung tissue, with the heart and great vessels taking up a large area as well.

Respiratory System

- *Pneumothorax.* Presence of air in the pleural cavity where the lung tissue has collapsed; a disruption of visceral pleura
- *Hemothorax.* Presence of blood in the pleural cavity
- *Central bronchogenic carcinoma.* Cancer in and around the hilum area of the mediastinum
- *Peripheral bronchogenic carcinoma.* Cancer in and around the bronchioles
- *Fibrous histiocytoma.* Granulomatous infiltration of interstitial by nonneoplastic histiocytes; common in young men; disease will regress
- *Pneumonia.* Inflammation of the lungs
- *Pulmonary edema.* Balance between capillary pressure and plasma pressure is lost with a build-up of fluid in the lungs
- *Metastasis.* Most common lung neoplasm; 80% from breast, skeletal, or renal primaries

Cardiovascular System

- *Cardiomegaly.* Enlargement of the heart
- *Aortic aneurysm.* Ballooning of vessel caused by disease or weakening for other reasons
- *Aortic dissection.* Intimal tear in wall of vessel creating two paths for blood to flow; created under high pressure; blood dissects layers of smooth muscles
- *Carditis.* Inflammation of the lining of the heart
- *Pulmonary embolism.* Obstruction of artery going to the lungs
- *Thrombus.* Formed from different components of blood (platelets, red blood cells, white blood cells); causes blockage in vessels

CHAPTER 7

Computed Tomography of the Abdomen

Chapter at a glance

INTRODUCTION TO BASIC PROTOCOLS

Computed tomography (CT) of the abdomen is similar to chest CT, using the spiral breath-hold technique. Better visualization of the organs and vessels is accomplished. Intravenous (IV) and oral contrasts are used routinely in preparation for CT abdominal scanning. Peritoneal and retroperitoneal structures are important for the technologists. A standard protocol follows as an example for abdomen imaging in Table 7-1.

TABLE 7-1	Standard Abdominal Protocol	
COMPONENT	CHEMICAL
Routine abdomen (standard)	Anterior to posterior scout (7 mm from top of diaphragm down to symphysis pubis) mAs = 330 kVp = 120 Matrix = 256 × 256 DFOV = 400 mm Routinely with oral and IV contrast (pressure injector)

DFOV, Display field of view; *IV,* intravenous; *kVp,* kilovolts peak; *mAs,* milli-amperes per second.

Strategic Anatomy

Similar to the chest, several important structures can be scanned to properly diagnosis abdominal problems. These structures range from bony components to the numerous organs found in the peritoneal and retroperitoneal cavities of the abdomen.

Bony Anatomy
- Ribs
- Thoracic and lumbar vertebrae

Surface Muscles
- *Transverse abdominis.* Most external
- *External oblique.* Middle layer
- *Internal oblique.* Most internal
- *Linea alba.* Tendinous membrane where three muscles converge anteriorly

Interior Muscles
- *Diaphragm.* Inferior extensions into abdominal cavity called crura (attached to lumbar vertebrae)
- *Rectus abdominis.* Either side of midline from crest of the pubis to xiphoid process
- *Psoas.* Originates from transverse processes of lumbar vertebrae; inserts at lesser trochanter

- ■ *Iliacus.* Inner aspect of the iliac crest; inserts into the lesser trochanter
- ■ *Quadratus lumborum.* Posterior abdominal wall

Abdominal Cavity

- ■ *Parietal peritoneum.* Serous membrane that lines the wall of abdominal cavity; liver, stomach transverse colon, spleen, ascending portion of duodenum, jejunum, ileum, and upper end of rectum, uterus, ovaries
- ■ *Visceral peritoneum.* Covering organs protruding through wall
- ■ *Peritoneal spaces.* Right and left subphrenic; right and left subhepatic; Morison's pouch, which is the deepest and where fluid easily collects; right and left paracolic gutters where free fluid will collect
- ■ *Retroperitoneum.* Behind the peritoneum; kidneys, pancreas, duodenum, ascending and descending portions of colon
- ■ *Retroperitoneal spaces.* Anterior and posterior pararenal space; perirenal space

Liver

- ■ *Largest organ.* Sits in right upper quadrant
- ■ Metabolic regulation, hematologic regulation, bile production
- ■ *Lobes*
  - ❑ *Caudate.* Medial, superior, posterior
  - ❑ *Quadrate,* Medial, inferior, anterior
  - ❑ *Right.* Occupies right hypochondriac region
  - ❑ *Left.* Extends occasionally over midline and sits anterior
- ■ *Falciform ligament.* Thin anteroposterior fold of peritoneum attaching to convex surface of liver, diaphragm, anterior abdominal wall
- ■ *Ligamentum venosum* (ductus venosus in fetal circulation). Separates left lobe from caudate lobe
- ■ *Ligamentum teres.* Separates quadrate lobe from right lobe
- ■ *Inferior vena cava.* Separates caudate lobe from right lobe

- **Gallbladder.** Separates quadrate lobe from right lobe
- **Porta hepatis.** Where blood vessels enter and exit the liver on its inferior surface
- **Portal hepatic system.** Flow of blood from digestive organs to liver before returning to heart
  - ❑ *Hepatic artery.* Delivers oxygenated blood to liver
  - ❑ *Hepatic portal vein.* Delivers deoxygenated blood from the digestive organs

The liver monitors substances before they are sent to the heart for general circulation. The superior mesenteric, inferior mesenteric, and the splenic veins drain into the hepatic portal vein. The hepatic portal system of veins drains the blood from the pancreas, spleen, stomach, intestines, and gallbladder. These veins are composed of the superior mesenteric, splenic, pancreatic, inferior mesenteric, and cystic veins.

The hepatic artery, vein, and duct comprise the hepatic triad. The hepatic ducts drain bile from liver. The right and left join to form the common hepatic duct. The cystic duct drains the gallbladder. The common bile duct is formed from the cystic and common hepatic duct.

Gallbladder

The *gallbladder,* which lies at the level of the ninth coastal cartilage on the inferior surface of the liver, is a saclike reservoir for bile along the right edge of the quadrate lobe of the liver. Parts of the gallbladder include the fundus, body, and neck. The bile empties into the cystic duct.

Pancreas

The *pancreas* is an elongated gland with endocrine and exocrine functions. Endocrine functions include the production of insulin and glucagon; exocrine functions produce pancreatic juice. This organ sits in the retroperitoneal, lying across the posterior surface of the abdomen from the duodenum to the spleen. The head of the pancreas lies within the curve of the duodenum continuing into the uncinate process. The neck is the constricted portion of the pancreas to the left of the head. The body extends to the left and sits superiorly across the aorta. The tail is the most posterior and superior portion of the pancreas.

Wirsung's duct begins in the tail, runs through the gland, and empties into the duodenum. The pancreas has a distinct lobulated appearance on the CT image.

Spleen

The *spleen* is a highly vascular organ that lies posteriorly to the stomach and is closely related to the left kidney and transverse colon. The tail of the pancreas sits close to the hilum of the spleen, which is the largest mass of lymphatic tissue. The circulation is provided by the splenic artery and vein, which enter and exit at the hilum between the gastric and renal depressions. The spleen filters abnormal blood cells, stores iron, and initiates immune response.

Adrenal Glands

The *adrenal glands* sit bilaterally on the upper border of the kidneys. The left gland appears Y-shaped, and the right gland is a triangular-shaped structure. The adrenal is an endocrine gland producing epinephrine, norepinephrine, mineralocorticoids, and glucocorticoids, the functions of which affect all of the body systems.

Kidneys

The right and left *kidneys* lie in the retroperitoneal cavity adjacent to the vertebral column, approximately T12 through L3. The hilum of the kidney is the medial indented region where the blood vessels enter and exit the kidney, as well as where the ureters exit the kidneys. The cortex is the outer region of the kidneys, which filters urine. The inner region, known as the medulla, is the collecting system. The renal fascia (perirenal fat) is Gerota's fascia, which anchors the kidneys. The calyceal system collects urine and drains into the renal pelvis and then into the ureter. The ureters then travel inferiorly and medially along the psoas muscle. The renal artery (from the aorta) and vein provide circulation. The left renal vein is longer than the right renal vein and crosses anterior to the aorta. When viewing a contrasted CT scan of the kidney, the renal vein is the most anterior vascular structure in the hilum, with the renal artery being in the middle and the urine filled ureter the most posterior.

Stomach

The anterior surface of the *stomach* involves the diaphragm, the left lobe of the liver, and the anterior abdominal wall. The posterior surface of the stomach involves the spleen, left kidney, adrenal gland, pancreas, and transverse colon. The lesser curvature of the stomach is directed to the right and superiorly and is continuous with the right margin of the esophagus. The cardiac orifice is where the esophagus enters the stomach at about the seventh costal cartilage. The pylorus is the lower portion of the stomach, which empties into the duodenum. The stomach extends from TII to LI.

Small Intestines

The mesentery is a double-walled sheet of peritoneum covering the *small intestines*. The duodenum curves around the head of the pancreas and is divided into four parts:

- **First part.** Superior part is horizontal, from pylorus to the gallbladder
- **Second part.** Turns sharply downward along posterior abdominal wall where pancreatic and bile ducts enter
- **Third part.** Inferior and horizontal, extends across midline, passing anterior to the inferior vena cava, aorta, right ureter, right gonadal vessels, psoas
- **Fourth part.** Ascends to the left of the aorta

The jejunum of the small intestine is a highly coiled tube located in the umbilical region of the abdomen, most of which lies in the hypogastric region and terminates in the right iliac region by an opening in the cecum (ileocecal valve). The ileum of the small intestine lies mainly in the hypogastric and pelvic regions.

Large Intestines

The cecum, into which the small intestine drains, is located in the right iliac region. The colon is divided into four parts:

- **Ascending.** Passes superiorly on the right side towards the liver to the hepatic flexure along the posterior abdominal wall
- **Transverse.** Passes across the abdomen to the splenic flexure; most superior portion

- **Descending.** Passes downward from the splenic flexure to the iliac crest
- **Sigmoid.** Begins at the iliac crest, crosses the sacrum, and curves to the midline at S-3
- **Rectum.** Point of origin and extends below the coccyx and becomes the anal canal

Vasculature

The aorta sits retroperitoneal and bifurcates into right and left iliac arteries.

- **Unpaired branches of the aorta**
  - ❑ *Celiac.* First branch arises near L-1; gives rise to common hepatic, splenic, gastric arteries
  - ❑ *Superior mesenteric.* Arises ventrally near L1 and L2, travels downward and to the right; supplies small intestine, excluding the duodenum, cecum, ascending and transverse colon
  - ❑ *Inferior mesenteric.* Arises ventrolaterally at L-3, travels downward and to the left; supplies distal transverse, descending, sigmoidal, and rectal portions of the colon
  - ❑ *Medial sacral.* Arises from posterior surface of the aorta, proximal to the bifurcation of the aorta; produces a pair of lumbar arteries
- **Paired branches of the aorta**
  - ❑ *Adrenal.* Small arteries that arise from the aorta at the level of the superior mesenteric artery, traveling laterally and superiorly to each adrenal gland
  - ❑ *Renal.* Two larger arteries that arise from sides of the aorta at L-2 and travel laterally to enter the hilum of the kidney; right renal artery is slightly longer than the left and passes posterior to the inferior vena cava, right renal vein, pancreatic head, and second part of the duodenum; left renal artery lies posterior to the body of the pancreas, left renal vein, and splenic vein
  - ❑ *Gonadal.* Arises below the renal arteries and descend through the abdomen to supply the gonads (ovarian and testicular)

❑ *Gonadal veins.* Ascend anteriorly to ureters to drain into inferior vena cava and renal vein

❑ *Lumbar.* Four pairs arise from the posterolateral surface of the aorta to supply the posterolateral abdominal wall

❑ *Lumbar veins.* Four or five pairs; some of which drain into the inferior vena cava and others into the azygos system

■ Inferior vena cava and tributaries

❑ *Inferior vena cava.* Largest vein; formed by junction of the right and left common iliac veins anterior to L-5; lies to the right of the aorta

❑ *Common iliac, renal, right adrenal, inferior phrenic, and hepatic veins.* Drain into the inferior vena cava

Specific Protocols

An anteroposterior (AP) scout of the abdomen is acquired with the patient in the supine position (Table 7-2). The scans are set up to cover the region of the body between the level of the diaphragm and the level of the iliac crest. Respiration is suspended for each scan unless spiral is used. Spiral is recommended because of the indication for IV contrast for all routine scans of the abdomen and pelvis. Oral contrast is given several hours ahead of time to opacify the bowel. A cup of oral contrast is given immediately before the scan to visualize the stomach. Routine abdomen scans are performed at 7 mm slice thicknesses with a field of view of 400 mm. (Refer to protocol at beginning of this chapter.)

Trauma abdomen protocols are generally set up to visualize any blunt trauma to the liver, kidneys, diaphragm, and pancreas. IV and oral contrast are required. A splenic injury may not be revealed for days. Diaphragmatic rupture can cause a herniation of abdominal organs in the chest. The pancreas is protected but

Table 7-2   Contrast Rates for Abdominal CT

ROUTINE DELAY TIMES FOR CONTRASTING THE ABDOMEN	
Flow rate: 2.0–2.5 cc/sec (150 cc total contrast)	10–20 second delay before scan start

can be injured with blunt trauma from a steering wheel of a car or bicycle handlebars. In the kidneys, coagulated hematomas are best visualized without an IV contrast. Lacerations, fractures of organs, and any vascular injury are best viewed with contrast. Renal, pelvic, calyceal, and uretal injuries are best viewed with a contrast delay (Figures 7-1 and 7-2).

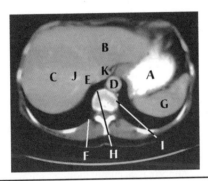

Figure 7-1 **Axial CT view of the abdomen.** *A,* Stomach; *B,* left lobe of liver; *C,* right lobe of liver; *D,* descending aorta; *E,* inferior vena cava; *F,* erector spinae muscle; *G,* spleen; *H,* azygos vein; *I,* hemiazygos vein; *J,* hepatic triad; *K,* caudate lobe of liver.

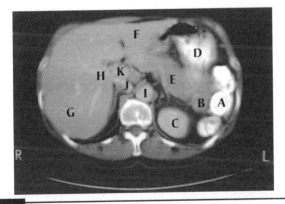

Figure 7-2 **Axial CT view of the abdomen.** *A,* Descending colon; *B,* bowel; *C,* right kidney; *D,* stomach; *E,* pancreas; *F,* left lobe of liver; *G,* right lobe of liver; *H,* portal vein; *I,* descending aorta; *J,* right adrenal gland; *K,* inferior vena cava.

When scanning the adrenal glands or pancreas specifically, 4 to 5 mm slice thicknesses are obtained. Spiral scanning can be used with special windowing of the images. Kidney CT scans are obtained before and after contrast. The cortex will enhance first and then the inner medulla. For a kidney stone protocol, smaller slice thicknesses are used with no contrast. Contrast blocks the visualization of the stone.

When scanning the liver, a bolus of contrast is given. Immediately after contrast, liver lesions appear hypodense. With a short delay, the lesions become isodense with the liver; with a longer delay, they will eventually become hyperdense.

COMMON ABNORMALITIES OF THE ABDOMEN

- **Hemorrhage.** Gray fluid viewing the abdominal cavity (blood)
- **Lymphoma.** Lymph node enlargement; 80% non-Hodgkin's
- **Ascites.** Abnormal accumulation of serous fluid in the peritoneal cavity; a result of numerous disorders
- **Retroperitoneal tumors.** Become extremely large, heterogenous components; liposarcoma is an example
- **Peritonitis.** Inflammation of peritoneal cavity; caused by leaking of perforated bowel
- **Portal hypertension.** Obstruction of blood flow in the portal hepatic system; can cause ascites or splenomegaly
- **Pancreatitis.** Inflammation of the pancreas, calcification, "ratty" appearance; leakage of powerful digestive enzymes, which will "digest" tissue
- **Pseudocysts.** Fluid-filled thus darker; occur in the pancreas
- **Gallbladder cancer.** Adenocarcinoma; squamous cell, calcified, or "porcelain" gallbladder
- **Gastric cancer.** Occurs most often in Japan; mucosa (lining of stomach) is ulcerated
- **Esophageal cancer.** Squamous cell adenocarcinoma, intraluminal mass
- **Hemochromatosis.** Disorder of iron metabolism with excess deposition of iron in tissues; bronze skin pigmentation; cirrhosis of liver, diabetes

- **Renal artery stenosis.** Renal ischemia; usually from hypertension
- **Renal cell carcinoma.** 85% of renal tumors; infiltrates the inferior vena cava through renal vein
- **Polycystic disease.** Vast enlargement of the kidneys with numerous cysts; hereditary disease
- **Cystic nephroma.** Cystic lesion not extending beyond cortical margin of kidney; composed of neural tissue
- **Hemangioma.** Vascular lesion
- **Hepatoma.** Liver lesion
- **Fatty liver.** From hypodense to normal liver tissue
- **Cirrhosis.** Liver disease characterized by loss of normal lobular architecture; fibrous bands of connective tissue form, constrict, and partition liver into irregular nodules
- **Liver metastasis.** Lesions from breast cancer, lung cancer, or melanoma; necrotic dark components on CT
- **Liver laceration.** Tearing of liver tissue from trauma; bleeds into organ itself
- **Splenomegaly.** Enlargement of the spleen; secondary to portal hypertension; hemolytic disease of the blood can cause deposits of iron and calcium
- **Spleen infarction.** Ischemic condition from insufficient arterial supply or venous outflow; necrosis of tissue occurs
- **Hernia.** Protrusion of a sac of peritoneum through a defect or weakness in the abdominal wall

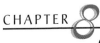
Computed Tomography of the Pelvis

Chapter at a glance

INTRODUCTION TO BASIC PROTOCOLS

This chapter should be viewed as a continuation of Chapter 7. Routinely, the pelvis is scanned with the abdomen (Table 8-1), which is performed to assess the extent of tumor involvement into the organs and to document treatment success or failure. A routine pelvis protocol will mimic a protocol for the abdomen. Intravenous (IV) and oral contrasts are used.

STRATEGIC ANATOMY

In this chapter, the bony anatomy and organs of the pelvis will be highlighted. In addition, male and female organs of the pelvis will be reviewed.

Bony Anatomy

- **Sacrum.** Lower portion of spine
- **Coccyx.** Three to five small fused bones
- **Ilium.** Body and large winglike projections; crest gives rise to superior and inferior iliac spines

TABLE 8-1	Pelvis Protocol
PROTOCOL	DESCRIPTION
Routine pelvis (standard)	Usually performed with routine abdomen protocol
	Anterior to posterior scout (7 mm from top of diaphragm down to symphysis pubis)
	mAs = 330
	kVp = 120
	Matrix = 256 × 256
	DFOV = 400 mm
	Usually with oral and IV contrast (pressure injector)
	Female pelvis: tampon used to visualize vaginal vault (clinical site-dependent)

DFOV, Display field of view; *IV*, intravenous; *kVp*, kilovolts peak; *mAs*, milli-amperes per second.

- *Pubis.* Body plus superior and inferior public rami; bodies meet to form symphysis pubis
- *Ischium.* Body plus two rami: ischial tuberosity and ischial spine

Pelvic Muscles

- *Extra pelvic*
  - ❏ Rectus abdominis, psoas, internal and external obliques
  - ❏ Rotation of spine and compression of abdominal and pelvic viscera
- *Muscles of the hip (gluteales)*
  - ❏ *Maximus.* Largest; most external
  - ❏ *Medius.* Middle layer
  - ❏ *Minimus.* Innermost layer
  - ❏ All of these muscles sit on the posterior aspect of the ilium
- *Pelvic wall muscles*
  - ❏ *Piriformis.* Pear-shaped muscle; rotates thigh
  - ❏ *Obturator internus and externus.* Moves thigh laterally and medially
  - ❏ *Iliacus.* Lines the iliac fossa

- ❏ *Iliopsoas.* Joining of the psoas and iliacus; flexion of leg
- ■ *Pelvic diaphragm muscles*
  - ❏ *Funnel-shaped muscles.* Make up the pelvic floor
  - ❏ *Levator ani.* Largest of pelvic floor; provides support for pelvic contents
  - ❏ *Coccygeus.* Posterior portion of pelvic floor; also provides support

Pelvic Organs

- ■ *Urinary bladder*
  - ❏ Distensible muscular organ; rests on the pelvic floor when empty; superior surface covered by peritoneum
  - ❏ Reservoir for storage of urine
  - ❏ Three openings called trigone; two for ureters, one for urethra
- ■ *Female urethra.* Short muscular tube; drains urine to outside of body through an opening anterior to the vagina
- ■ *Male urethra.* Three parts; prostatic, membranous, penile

Female Pelvis and Male Pelvis

- ■ *Female.* Peritoneum reflected onto the anterior wall of the uterus to form the vesicouterine pouch
- ■ *Rectouterine pouch.* Sits between the uterus and rectum
- ■ *Male.* Peritoneum reflected onto the rectum and is called the rectovesical pouch
- ■ *Rectum*
  - ❏ Originates at the level of S3; 12 cm in length; becomes the anal canal
  - ❏ Terminal part of large intestine

Female Pelvis

- ■ *Ovaries*
  - ❏ Sit in the ovarian fossa, which is a shallow depression in the lateral wall of the pelvis; position can vary greatly; supported by suspensory ligaments
  - ❏ *Suspensory ligaments:* Round, uterosacral, lateral cervical
- ■ *Fallopian tubes.* Lateral to the uterus, supported by the broad ligament

- **_Uterus_**
  - ❑ Hollow, muscular, pear-shaped organ
  - ❑ Located in the anterior portion of the pelvic cavity, above the vagina and between the rectum and bladder
  - ❑ Wall has three layers—endometrium, myometrium, perimetrium; receives the embryo resulting from a fertilized egg
  - ❑ Suspensory ligaments also stabilize the uterus
- **_Vagina._** Extends from cervix of uterus to external vaginal orifice

Male Pelvis

- **_Prostate_**
  - ❑ Largest accessory gland of the male reproductive system; located inferior to the bladder
  - ❑ Surrounds the prostatic urethra, which is located below the bladder between the pubis and rectum
- **_Testes_**
  - ❑ Primary reproductive organs of the male; suspended in a sac of skin called the scrotum
  - ❑ Produce sperm and male sex hormones
  - ❑ Transmit sperm to epididymis where sperm mature
- **_Vas deferens_**
  - ❑ Continuation of epididymis; joins with duct of seminal vesicle to form ejaculatory duct
  - ❑ Each vas deferens is surrounded by spermatic cords
  - ❑ Tubular structures travel from the testicle through the inguinal canal to the fundus of the bladder, curls around the bladder and enters the posterior aspect of the prostate
- **_Seminal vesicles_**
  - ❑ Small lobules sitting against the posterior bladder wall; accessory gland; superior to prostate
  - ❑ Secrete seminal fluid that mixes with sperm before ejaculation
- **_Penis_**
  - ❑ External male reproductive organ
  - ❑ Composed of erectile tissue

Vasculature

- Aorta bifurcates into the common iliacs at L4 (Figure 8-1)

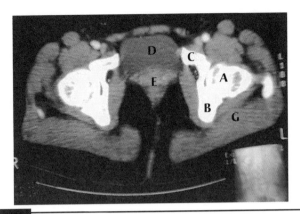

Figure 8-1 Aorta bifurcates into the common iliacs at L4. *A,* Femoral head; *B,* ischium; *C,* pubic bone; *D,* bladder; *E,* prostate; *G,* gluteal muscle.

- Common iliacs branch into the internal and external iliac arteries at the lumbosacral junction
- The external iliac becomes the femoral artery
- Femoral veins course back through the external iliac vein, which drains into the common iliac vein, which in turn drains into the inferior vena cava near L5
- *Sciatic nerve*
  - Part of sacral plexus
  - Enters posterior gluteal region via sciatic notch
  - Travels into left lateral to ischial tuberosity
- *Lymph nodes*
  - Around the iliac arteries, obturator internus muscle, sacrum
  - Inguinal ligament lies between the anterior superior iliac spine (ASIS) and pubis

SPECIFIC PROTOCOLS

The patient is supine and an AP scout is acquired to set up the scans. As previously noted, CT scans of the pelvis and abdomen are routinely acquired together. Slice thicknesses are usually 7 mm and spiral scanning is used. The pelvic part of spiral may be delayed for the IV contrast to have time to reach the bladder for visualization. (Refer to Table 7-2 for contrast rate.)

Common Abnormalities of the Pelvis

Several types of disease affect organs in the female and male pelvis. Different diseases can strike the sexes and many are diagnosed and followed up with CT scanning.

- **Pheochromocytoma.** Adrenal gland tumor causing excessive production of epinephrine and norepinephrine
- **Cushing's disease.** Excess of free-circulating cortisol from the adrenal cortex; buffalo hump; moon face characteristics
- **Bladder cancer.** Transitional cell; multiple filling defects in bladder with usual dilation of one ureter; mass surrounded by contrast; hematuria, pain
- **Ovarian cancer.** Leading cause of death from gynecological cancers for women 40 to 65 years of age; epithelial cell is the most common
- **Endometrial cancer**
  - ❏ Most common invasive malignancy of female genital tract
  - ❏ Endometrial thickness
  - ❏ Perimenopausal or postmenopausal women
  - ❏ Associated with estrogen therapy
- **Prostate cancer**
  - ❏ Second most common cancer in men in the United States
  - ❏ CT is best modality
  - ❏ Involvement beyond gland into pelvic area
- **Seminoma.** Malignant tumor of the testes arising from germ cells; a testicular cancer
- **Testicular cancer**
  - ❏ Men 15 to 45 years of age
  - ❏ 90% is germ cell
  - ❏ Seminoma is the most common
  - ❏ Tumors painless; hardened by palpation

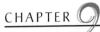
Musculoskeletal Computed Tomography

Chapter at a glance

INTRODUCTION TO BASIC PROTOCOLS

The area of musculoskeletal computed tomography (CT) involves imaging specific upper and lower extremity joints. Generally, CT is used for problem solving after a diagnostic x-ray is obtained. Useful protocols are found in Box 9-1. CT can help localize bony tumors and verify their extent into the cortical bone and the articular region. CT is especially useful with fractures to reveal orientation and relationships of fracture fragments to neurovascular or muscular components. Special software programs of multiplanar reconstruction (MPR) and three-dimensional (3-D) imaging are now available for this procedure. Intravenous (IV) contrast can also help determine relationships of tumors to tissues. The injection of an intraarticular contrast may also help with diagnosis.

STRATEGIC ANATOMY: UPPER EXTREMITIES

CT of the extremities is difficult because every bone or joint space must be scanned differently. The anatomy of the upper and lower extremities will be reviewed, with special emphasis on joints.

Shoulder

The shoulder is a ball-and-socket joint consisting of the clavicle, scapula, and humerus. The acromioclavicular (AC) joint is also a part of the shoulder region. The clavicle extends transversely from sternum to acromion of scapula to form the AC joint. The triangular-shaped scapula is composed of the spine, acromion, coracoid process, and the glenoid process. The glenoid process ends in a depression called the glenoid fossa, which is the attachment site for the humeral head. The bicipital groove is the attachment site for numerous tendons and ligaments. Separated by the bicipital groove, the lesser tubercle and greater tubercle comprise part of the humerus and provide attachment sites for tendons and ligaments. Bursa—synovial-filled sacs acting as buffers—surround all joints. The subacromial and the subdeltoid bursa are the largest in the body.

- ■ *Shoulder muscles.* The deltoid muscle surrounds the entire shoulder area. The rotator cuff is composed of the tendons of the infraspinatus, subscapularis, supraspina-

---

Box 9-1   Extremity CT Protocols

- ■ Tailored protocols, depending on extremity or joint to be imaged
- ■ Usually on bilateral joints for comparison (symmetry)
- ■ Thinner slice thicknesses
- ■ Smaller field of view
- ■ Soft tissue and bone windowing to visualize muscle-tissue versus bone
- ■ Algorithm (bone or detail)
- ■ Intravenous contrast possible
- ■ Intraarticular contrast possible

tus, and teres minor. The subscapularis is the only anterior tendon. The supraspinatus is the most frequently injured tendon. The biceps tendon is used for support of the shoulder. Magnetic resonance imaging (MRI) is preferred for rotator cuff tears and for other injuries involving the shoulder. CT is obtained for bony problems.

- *Labrum and ligaments*
    - ❑ *Glenoid labrum*
    - ❑ *Fibrocartilaginous ring.* Deepens the articular surface of the glenoid fossa; glenohumeral ligaments contribute to the formation of the glenoid labrum
    - ❑ *Coracoacromial ligament.* Protects humeral head and rotator cuff tendons from direct trauma
    - ❑ *Coracoclavicular ligament.* Maintains position of clavicle

Elbow

- *Humerus*
    - ❑ Distal portion of the humerus has a medial condyle and lateral condyle with associated epicondyles
    - ❑ Two depressions located on distal humerus; coronoid fossa and olecranon fossa
    - ❑ Articular surface of distal humerus are capitellum and trochlea
- *Radius.* Radial head is flattened; articulates with capitellum of humerus and radial notch of ulna
- *Ulna.* Proximal ulna contains the olecranon and coronoid processes; large trochlea notch, which articulates with humerus
- *Ligaments of elbow*
    - ❑ *Ulnar collateral.* Reinforces medial side of elbow
    - ❑ *Radial ulnar collateral.* Reinforces lateral side of elbow
    - ❑ *Annular ligament.* Binds radial head to radial notch of ulna
- *Muscles*
    - ❑ *Anterior group.* Brachialis and biceps brachii (flexors of forearm)
    - ❑ *Posterior group.* Triceps brachii (main extensor of forearm) and anconeus (pronates ulna)
    - ❑ *Lateral group.* Brachioradialis; extensor muscles of fingers and wrist; supinator

- ❑ *Medial.* Pronator teres; flexor muscles of fingers and wrist
- ■ *Vasculature*
  - ❑ Brachial artery bifurcates into radial and ulnar at cubital fossa
  - ❑ Median cubital vein creates a joining of basilic and cephalic veins, which are tributaries of axillary vein
- ■ *Ulnar nerve.* Between the medial epicondyle of the humerus and the olecranon process; most frequently injured

Wrist

- ■ Composed of the distal radius, ulna, and eight carpal bones
- ■ *Eight carpal bones.* Scaphoid, triquetral, trapezium, capitate, lunate, pisiform, trapezoid, hamate
- ■ Radius and ulna each have a styloid process
- ■ Carpal tunnel in the wrist is the concave arrangement of the carpal bones through which the median nerve traverses
- ■ Palmar tendons of the wrist are responsible for flexion
- ■ Dorsal tendons are responsible for extension
- ■ Triangular fibrocartilage is the stabilizing element of the wrist joint; located on the radial side of the wrist
- ■ Ulnar artery courses with the ulnar nerve
- ■ Radial artery courses with the median nerve

Sternum

- ■ An elongated flat bone; not a joint
- ■ Composed of three parts: manubrium, body, xiphoid
- ■ Clavicles articulate with the manubrium
- ■ First seven ribs articulate with the sternum
- ■ Fractures or injuries to the sternum occur most often in automobile accidents or other types of trauma

STRATEGIC ANATOMY: LOWER EXTREMITIES

Pelvic Girdle-Hip

- ■ *Acetabulum.* Cavity created by ilium, ischium, and pubis; attachment site for the femoral head

■ Acetabular fossa is a nonarticulating depression within the acetabulum
■ *Femur.* Fovea capitis
  ❏ Small pit located on head of femur
  ❏ Route for transmission of blood vessels to the femoral head
■ *Ligaments of the hip*
  ❏ *Acetabular labrum.* Creates rim attached to margin of acetabulum; increases stability to hip joint
  ❏ *Transverse.* Inferior margin of acetabulum reinforced
  ❏ *Iliofemoral ligament.* Provides reinforcement to anterior portion of hip
■ *Muscles*
  ❏ *Anterior group.* Quadriceps femoris, iliopsoas, sartorius
  ❏ *Posterior.* Obturator internus-externus, quadriceps femoris, piriformis, superior-inferior gemellus
  ❏ *Medial.* Pectineus, adductor, gracilis
  ❏ *Lateral.* Three gluteal muscles (minimus, medius, maximum) and tensor fasciae latae
■ *Sciatic nerve.* Largest peripheral nerve of the body
■ *Femoral artery and vein.* Provide circulation

Knee
■ Hinged joint with a gliding motion (Figure 9-1)
■ *Bony components.* Femur, tibia, patella
■ Medial and lateral condyles and epicondyles
■ *Tibial plateaus.* Structures articulating surfaces of the tibia
■ *Tibial tuberosity.* Located on anterior surface; insertion site for patellar ligament
■ *Tibial spine.* Serves as attachment site for ligaments
■ *Patella.* Protects anterior joint surface of knee; increases leverage of quadriceps muscle
■ Extremely fibrous capsule
■ *Menisci.* Concave cushion pads between the femoral condyle and tibial plateau
■ *Ligaments*
  ❏ Five intracapsular and extracapsular ligaments to strengthen the capsule

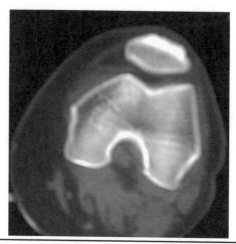

Figure 9-1 Axial CT of the knee shows the patella.

- ❏ *Collateral ligaments.* Medial on tibial side to strengthen; lateral on fibular side to strengthen
- ❏ *Cruciate ligaments.* Anterior and posterior inside the knee capsule; provides anterior and posterior stability to the knee
- ❏ *Patellar ligament.* Continuation of quadriceps tendon; helps maintain position of patella within joint
- ■ *Muscles*
  - ❏ Quadriceps femoris
  - ❏ *Hamstring group.* Extensors of thigh and flexors of leg
  - ❏ Popliteus
  - ❏ *Gastrocnemius.* Spans posterior part of knee to insert on calcaneus via Achilles tendon
- ■ Popliteal artery and vein provide circulation
- ■ Great saphenous vein sits laterally; routinely used for vessel grafts in other parts of the body
- ■ Most knee injuries and pathologies are now diagnosed with MRI; tendons and ligaments are easily visualized

Ankle and Foot

- ■ The ankle and foot form a hingelike joint with plantar and dorsi flexion (Figure 9-2)

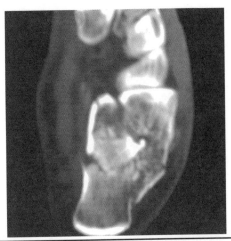

Figure 9-2 Axial CT of the foot shows fracture of the calcaneus.

- Articulations between the tibia, fibula, talus
- *Malleoli.* Prevent the medial (tibia) and lateral (fibula) displacement of the talus
- *Talus.* Articulates with tibia and fibula at ankle joint
- *Calcaneus.* Heel bone
- *Subtalar joint.* Formed with the calcaneus and talus
- *Tarsal bones.* Include the cuboid, navicular, and three cuneiform
- *Ligaments of the ankle*
  - *Deltoid ligaments.* Arise from medial malleolus expanding into tibiotalar, tibiocalcaneal, and tibiofibular ligaments
  - *Lateral ligaments.* Strengthen lateral border of ankle joint; anterior talofibular, calcaneofibular, posterior talofibular, anterior and posterior talofibular
  - *Plantar.* Maintain longitudinal arch of foot
  - *Interosseous.* Band of tissue binding talus to calcaneus
- *Tendons of the ankle*
  - *Posterior group.* Achilles tendon; arises from gastrocnemius and soleus; attaches to calcaneal tuberosity
  - *Anterior group*
    - Tibialis anterior

- Extensor hallucis longus
- Extensor digitorum longus
  ❑ *Medial group*
    - Posterior tibialis
    - Flexor digitorum
    - Flexor hallucis
  ❑ *Lateral group*
    - Peroneus longus
    - Peroneus brevis

COMMON BONY ABNORMALITIES OF THE MUSCULOSKELETAL SYSTEM

CT of the extremities is often performed during times of fractures to "put the pieces back together again." Most of the work involving ligaments and tumors is accomplished through MR scanning.

- **Tumors**
  ❑ *Osteochondroma.* Benign lesion; varies in size; occurs in the femur, tibia, pelvis
  ❑ *Osteosarcoma.* Malignant lesion; grows from bone tissue; relates to growth or repair
  ❑ *Lytic lesion.* Disruption of red blood cells in marrow
- **Avascular necrosis.** Subcapital fractures of femoral head; usually from disruption of arterial blood supply to area
- **Osteoporosis.** Decreased mass per unit volume of bone

References
Durham D: *Atlas of CT pathology.* Philadelphia: W.B. Saunders, 1977.
Kelly L, Peterson D: *Sectional anatomy for imaging professionals.* St. Louis: Mosby, 1997.
Seeram E: *Computed tomography physical principles clinical applications and quality control.* Philadelphia: W.B. Saunders, 1994.
Seeram E. Dose in CT. *Radiologic Technology.* 1998;70(6):534-556.
Seeram E: Review questions for CT. Malden, MA: Blackwell Science, 1997.
Scroggins D et al: *Lippincott's CT review.* Philadelphia: J.B. Lippincott, 1995.

Index